IMPROVING QUALITY IN HEALTHCARE

IMPROVING QUALITY IN HEALTHCARE

QUESTIONING THE WORK FOR EFFECTIVE CHANGE

MURRAY ANDERSON-WALLACE
NICK DOWNHAM

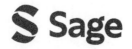

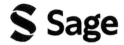

1 Oliver's Yard
55 City Road
London EC1Y 1SP

2455 Teller Road
Thousand Oaks, California 91320

Unit No 323-333, Third Floor, F-Block
International Trade Tower Nehru Place
New Delhi 110 019

8 Marina View Suite 43-053
Asia Square Tower 1
Singapore 018960

Editor: Laura Walmsley
Editorial Assistant: Sahar Jamfar
Production Editor: Neelu Sahu
Copyeditor: Tom Bedford
Indexer: Cathryn Pritchard
Marketing Manager: Ruslana Khatagova
Cover Design: Sheila Tong
Typeset by KnowledgeWorks Global Ltd
Printed and bound by
CPI Group (UK) Ltd, Croydon, CR0 4YY

Library of Congress Control Number: 2023938722

British Library Cataloguing in Publication data

A catalogue record for this book is available from the British Library

ISBN 978-1-5297-3306-8
ISBN 978-1-5297-3305-1 (pbk)

At Sage we take sustainability seriously. Most of our products are printed in the UK using responsibly sourced papers and boards. When we print overseas we ensure sustainable papers are used as measured by the Paper Chain Project grading system. We undertake an annual audit to monitor our sustainability.

Contents

List of Figures and Tables

Figures

Tables

About the Authors

Murray Anderson-Wallace has a clinical background in mental health services and psychological therapy and is trained in systemic approaches to counselling, consultation and supervision. He is a qualified groupwork practitioner, registered with the Institute of Group Analysis. Murray has an enduring interest in the social dynamics of organising and has spent much of his career tackling complex socio-cultural and ethical issues, including leading several large-scale independent reviews of care. Murray has provided strategic support to a wide range of national quality programmes and networks in the UK and abroad. He has taught at postgraduate level internationally and is a visiting professor at the Health Systems Innovation Lab at London South Bank University. Murray's practice also includes work as an independent editor, writer and broadcaster, producing media to stimulate debate about complex professional and ethical issues in healthcare. He is co-author of *Networks in Healthcare: Managing Complex Relationships* (2016) with Professor Becky Malby.

Nick Downham is a healthcare quality, systems thinking and organisational development specialist. He is committed to helping clinicians, other professionals and communities be their most impactful in helping people live good lives. He has a quality and industrial engineering background and has spent most of his career working in health and social care. Nick has shaped, and continues to shape, some of the largest and most enduring quality improvement programmes in the NHS. He is visiting teaching faculty at the Health Systems Innovation Lab at London South Bank University and works with front line teams, and their leaders at all levels, in healthcare services across primary and secondary care domestically and internationally.

Acknowledgements

First and foremost, we would like to thank our families – Annie, Em and Merren; Helen, Eve and Toby – for their support, patience, and encouragement as we researched and wrote this book. We couldn't have done it without you.

We would also like to acknowledge all our colleagues at the Health Systems Innovation Lab at London South Bank University, whose good humour, forbearance and critique has helped us to explore and develop the concepts that form this book. Also, our thanks go to the many Darzi Clinical Fellows, who over the years have been willing to test, critique and develop our ideas as part of their learning. Finally, we both need to acknowledge Uncle Charlie, without whom this book would never have been written.

Specific Acknowledgements from Nick

I would like to thank John Bicheno. It was meeting and learning from John that set me on my now two-decade plus path of questioning rather than accepting how work is done and organised. He is always humble and generous in sharing his expertise. I would also like to acknowledge Liz Ward, proud nurse and longtime collaborator who more than anyone has helped me understand the unsanitised, profound, upsetting and rewarding work of healthcare. I'd also like to thank Murray, co-author of this book and long time collaborator. I thank you for your time, wisdom, good grace and commitment to this work. Thanks also to Malcolm Anker, who has given his precious time to refine this writing. Finally, I would like to thank Prof. Becky Malby, who has provided me with unparalleled opportunities to think about and challenge the assumptions and traditions that shape our systems of work.

Specific Acknowledgements from Murray

I would like to specifically acknowledge Dr Christine Oliver, Chris Blantern, Dr Tom Boydell and Amynta Cardwell whose collegiate spirit and wisdom shaped my early thinking about relational practice and quality. I'd also like to thank my good friend and colleague Dr Suzanne Shale, whose scholarship helped me to understand the strange moral world of healthcare. I too want to thank Prof. Becky Malby, who I have worked with for many years. Our work together at the Centre for Innovation in Health Management at the University of Leeds cemented my partnership with Nick, which led to this book. I'd also like to thank Dr Rebecca Myers for her ongoing support and friendship. Our conversations help me to maintain a curious stance in a world that is too quick to accept simplicity and dualism over complexity and paradox. Finally, my thanks go to all the families who have generously shared their painful lived experiences of healthcare harm, teaching me lessons that I could not have learnt any other way. Special thanks in that regard go to colleagues Joanne Hughes and James Titcombe OBE.

1

Context

Framing

There is little doubt that the health and care system in the UK, like many around the world, is under intense pressure. Some would argue that the NHS is facing the most significant challenges in its history at precisely the time when the requirement to reshape care to meet need is greater than ever.

And as we consider people's lived experiences of healthcare - citizens and professionals - we quickly get a sense of huge variability; from people who tell of good, often excellent compassionate and expert care environments, alongside accounts of intractable quality problems, growing inequity in terms of access and outcome, poor working conditions and excruciating inefficiency and waste. These realities co-exist - all are true - and it can be understandably bewildering and worrying for those who use services, and certainly challenging for those who have responsibility for providing them.

The dominant narratives offered to explain the current context are well rehearsed and numerous. The list is long and includes the increasing demand driven by demographic change and an ageing population; the effects of the COVID-19 pandemic; underinvestment during a period of fiscal austerity; the lack of a long-term workforce strategy leading to chronic shortages of staff; the rising costs of providing care in a period of high inflation and low economic growth; vast expansion in medical and scientific knowledge; growing expectations from citizens; and the harsh realities, tensions and distortions driven by politicians and the media - these are all familiar parts of the story. Just as familiar are the so-called solutions to these problems; a narrative that normally boils down to a conversation about additional resourcing, injection of private sector "expertise", more money, and very often structural reform. These "solutions" are largely focused on increasing the capacity of the system as a response, as the logical reaction to rising demand. On the face of it those solutions make sense, and in some cases are entirely appropriate. However, in this book we also want to explore an alternative starting position, which argues that we should give as much - if not more - attention to reducing demand, in particular demand that is created by the way that the system works.

A central theme of this book is the notion of Failure Demand, which is defined as the work that is generated by the current system of work that does not create value for the end users (Seddon, 2008). Failure Demand drains precious capacity; it is wasteful and often creates extremely poor experiences for citizens and professionals alike. We argue that identifying and naming sources of Failure Demand and responding to them can have a significant impact for all concerned. Tellingly, the concept of Failure Demand is not particularly new, and it is not a straightforward matter. It requires a willingness to grapple with some of the complex practical, ethical and psychological issues that we believe have a profound shaping effect on the socio-cultural and operational context of healthcare. It also requires us to have a strong grasp on some of the more technical aspects of healthcare provision, especially understandings of unwarranted variation and how we use the resources we have in the most effective ways.

What Does the Book Explore?

As the title of this book suggests, our focus is three-fold. Firstly, we are keen to understand what is meant by the term "quality" in healthcare, including an exploration of some core concepts of quality; their history and meaning in a contemporary context.

Secondly, we invite you to "question the work" which means adopting a more inquiring approach to our long-held assumptions about the purpose and nature of healthcare. In short, this means examining how we know that we are even doing the right work before attempting to improve it. Of course, this immediately raises the question of who gets to define what is "right" and thus usefully draws our attention to critical issues of power, purpose, knowledge and risk at the outset. We think this is a particularly good thing.

Finally, we want to invite a critical re-examination of the dominant approaches to change that are frequently adopted in "quality" work, many of which have been imported, adapted and in some cases "cherry-picked" from thinking and practice rooted in scientific management. Instead, we want to explore the contribution that ideas and practices from a more inter-disciplinary perspective can bring, when woven together with some important – but often overlooked – aspects of quality thinking.

In exploring the improvement of quality in health services, we will be using the perspective of and drawing from examples of the English NHS extensively. This is not only because we have spent much of our careers working within or close to the NHS, but also because its scale means it has been subject to huge investment in programmes of quality and the resulting study and reflection. Because of this the NHS provides a valuable platform for observation and reflection that is useful beyond the NHS itself. We have also drawn on examples from other high-performing healthcare systems that we have personally studied and certainly view our conclusions as transferable and useful to other healthcare systems, with appropriate adaptations for context.

What Do We Mean By "Quality" in Healthcare?

As discussed in Chapter 2, notions of quality, and in particular methods for quality improvement in organisations, have their genesis in industrial contexts, and many of the key figures who influenced the ideas were firmly rooted in environments other than healthcare. Boaden et al. (2008) note that many developments in healthcare quality have been professionally led, and thus reflect the different traditions and ways of working within the healthcare professions. This has led to quite a wide range of definitions of quality, and a degree of "cherry-picking" in terms of approach, method and technique. We believe that this has led to some crucial elements of quality thinking having been lost in translation or marginalised due to their challenge to traditional organisational thinking or simply because of the time it takes to fully understand and contextualise them.

Throughout this book we have adopted the widely accepted multi-dimensional definition of clinical quality first set out by the Institute of Medicine report "Crossing the Quality Chasm" (IoM, 2001). The definition encompasses important notions of effectiveness, safety, personal experience, productivity and efficiency and is discussed in greater detail later in the book. It was subsequently refined in the 2008 Government White Paper "High Quality Care for All" (Britain & Darzi, 2008) including some references to the core leadership behaviours that might be needed to ensure "implementation, continuous improvement and measuring success".

We are also attracted by the definitions outlined by Avendis Donabedian – the so-called father of medical outcomes research. In his model Donabedian emphasises six dimensions of quality, which despite being developed almost 50 years ago, convey quite a contemporary sensibility (Donabedian, 1966). Critically, improving clinical quality is framed as serving a wider moral purpose of creating more equitable and responsive services, and ultimately better health outcomes for the population – a means to an end, rather than an end-in-itself – a principle that we will return to repeatedly.

- The way the practitioner manages the personal interaction with the patient
- Patient's own contribution to care
- Amenities of the settings where care is provided
- Facility in access to care
- Social distribution of access
- Social distribution of health improvements attributable to care

---

Figure 1.1 Donabedian's six dimensions of quality (adapted from Donabedian, 1966)

Is the Book about Quality Improvement?

Put simply, the answer is no. There are plenty of excellent texts and resources to support people to understand quality improvement, and we are not attempting to replicate them. Moreover, for more than 30 years quality improvement has been advocated as a method to improve outcomes, experience and costs within the healthcare environment (Berwick, 2019), and yet the question of whether quality improvement improves quality has proved surprisingly difficult to answer (Dixon-Woods, 2019). Indeed, for some, despite all efforts in this domain, system performance has stagnated, and meaningful sustained improvements have proved elusive (Braithwaite, 2018).

It is also not our intention to either attack or defend quality improvement but to explore its genesis and effects. That is not to say that our position is neutral, and we certainly challenge some of the narrow approaches derived from "cherry-picking" from industrial and business contexts that have informed a great deal of quality improvement practice in healthcare. We are certainly interested in how these ideas have been understood, used and adopted in practice, and the genesis of some of the problems faced are certainly worthy of consideration. Overall, we hope to hypothesise about how a more "quality-informed" lens might offer options for achieving a more responsive, equitable and affordable healthcare system in the future, but not by slavishly applying techniques.

What Does It Mean to "Question the Work"?

Central to this book is the notion of curious inquiry, an approach that rejects passive acceptance and encourages questions that challenge the work we do in healthcare.

This means not only examining the need for and the scale of the work, but also to better understand how the dominant ideologies and systems of meaning that create, and are created by the work constrain and/or enable the development of high-quality care. In short, we believe this requires a subtle but critical re-examination of epistemology and ontology (i.e., the theories we hold about our knowledge and the beliefs we have about the nature of being) and to explore how they silently shape our relationships; inform our decisions and drive our actions – operationally, strategically and in our daily lived experiences. We believe that engaging in this "questioning" process – as opposed to striving for pronouncements of certainty and control – should be central to 21st century healthcare practice, which is characterised by incredible complexity, fragmentation, plurality and rapid emergent change. Throughout this book we will propose principles and methods that we hope will make this curious enquiry easier and more effective.

How Do We Understand Change?

In our research for this book, we have also drawn on our extensive personal experience of working in and around issues of clinical quality in healthcare at a national, regional and local level over the past three decades. We have reflected upon and critiqued our own role in national and local quality work – especially in our shared experience of spreading quality improvements at scale within the English NHS. It is safe to say that what we bring is potage – as a wise former colleague would have it[1] – by this we mean that the wide experience that has shaped our thinking and practice is akin to a thick soup, which whilst delicious to eat (we hope) has ingredients that work together because of the blend and is not a result of a carefully followed recipe. We have drawn upon a wide body of multi-disciplinary literature, including management, industrial engineering, psychology, sociology, anthropology, ethics and philosophy. All have important ideas to contribute as we think critically about the current context and challenges. Based on our interpretation of the literature and own lived experience, we have concluded that there are three important questions to consider when it comes to change:

Firstly, do we understand "it" as predominantly something we must invoke in a static world, or is "it" something we can only hope to shape given the constantly dynamic conditions? Put another way, is change the constant and statis the temporary state, or do we think that change must be induced, created and managed? This is not a straightforward question, but your response is important because of the way it will influence the choices you make when it comes to a quality intervention. Associated with this is the position that you think improvement leaders take in the process. Are they miners, responsible for creating the system conditions, and then drilling down for root causes to be fixed, or are they travellers embedded within a complex matrix of meaning and action, active participants in an ongoing interactive emergent process?

The second question to consider is whether we think re-organisation or restructuring equals change. Alongside colleagues, we have over the course of our careers experienced the effects of multiple structural re-organisations, several enacted in the name of improving quality. These have ranged from the introduction of general management[2] (Griffiths, 1983) in the 1980s to the decentralisation of commissioning to local clinical groups; from the internal market – developed in the belief that competitive market forces would drive improvements in quality – to the current preference for collaborative, integrated care systems, where promoting population health and reducing health inequalities is highlighted. But whatever the focus of the re-organisation has been, and despite all the noble intentions – not to mention the huge investment of time, money and energy – the measurable gains in quality at scale appear to have been marginal and inconsistent at best (Bate, 1994; Dixon-Woods, 2019). Of course, we can all cite some notable exceptions to prove the rule, but these have tended to occur in boundaried environments where quality has been optimised in specific areas of practice, often only to push quality problems into other domains. Moreover, even in these areas many of the hard-won gains have proved to be unsustainable or fragile over time. Nevertheless, one could argue that these attempts were worthwhile, each contributing in an iterative sense to the broader matrix of experience that supports evolution. Whatever your opinion, most would agree that it has been hard to tackle the complex systemic issues that influence the quality of care, not least because of the highly dynamic conditions that characterise most modern healthcare. It is also worth reminding ourselves that in the NHS many of these conditions, which are often labelled as emergent and unpredictable, such as workforce shortages, changes in patterns of disease, shortages of personal protective equipment, lack of focus on proactive care – are often foreseen in detail with perfectly reasonable mitigation proposed ahead of time – it is just that they are not acted upon.

Thirdly, an important distinction to make right away is the distinction between things being complex and being complicated. When things are complex, we experience possibility, change and messiness, but these do not always elicit difficulty. Complexity requires us to draw on our relational skills and sensibilities, sometimes temporarily simplifying things to hold the complexity at the same time, but never atomising or breaking down into component parts. In contrast, complicated problems necessitate a greater application of technical knowledge and frequently benefit from being broken down into smaller parts.

When things are complicated, they are often difficult to solve and may require a significant amount of time and effort, but they are addressable with the proper knowledge, rules and recipes.

Complex issues rarely have simple solutions and necessitate flexibility, adaptation, iteration and innovation to move forward. The goal in this domain is to try to connect things and to see people and organisations as relational realities that emerge from local interaction rather than as separate entities. Stability and change are thus viewed as relational processes, with power understood as moral and communal, with ethics at the centre. This approach prioritises processes of inquiry, reflection, challenge and critique, but always in the service of a collaborative task. It acknowledges the need to hold the complexity of our situations, even when we may choose to temporarily simplify for the sake of acting, and to learn to live with uncertainty and the unknown. This can produce anxiety in ourselves and in others, which needs to be acknowledged and supported if we are to avoid the unhelpful and sometimes toxic effects of suppressing these very real issues.

A framework that we have found helpful in this regard defines three modes of organising and thus to the way we approach change. Each has its own legitimacy, which is defined not by any inherent value, but rather through an understanding of its utility in a specific context. The third mode – which is described as "relational" or "systemic" – claims to offer specific promise for conditions where complexity, fragmentation, distributed knowledge and power are present. Choosing when to adopt one approach or another is therefore important, and part of the relational leadership task (Anderson-Wallace et al., 2001a; Anderson-Wallace et al., 2001b; Malby & Anderson-Wallace, 2016).

Mode 1: Mechanistic: "Doing things well" – The emphasis here is on control. This mode of operation relies on "recipe-tradition" based current practice to ensure consistency and reliability within accepted routines. Power and knowledge are centralised. This mode does not respond to changes in environment, and people tend to be viewed as human resources that can be trained to reproduce consistent behaviour. The dominant mode of communication is transactional and involves repeating simple messages reliably over time. Governance is based on a compliance model, which requires effecting policing, usually by managers. Scientific management arising from Taylorism is the dominant ideology. Leading quality thinker, and one of the three big quality gurus of our time,[3] Joseph Juran, defines this mode as the phase of Quality Control in his Quality Trilogy (Juran, 1989). This focuses on the meeting of established goals, the detection of departures from planned levels of performance and the restoration of performance to the planned levels (Juran, 1989, p. 145). In an important departure from the NHS's top-down approach to quality control, to police or scrutinise, Juran details the hierarchy of control from most to least impactful as automated controls, control by the workforce, control by supervisors and managers and finally control by upper managers (Juran, 1989, p. 148).

Mode 2: Participative: "Doing things better" – The emphasis here is on improving. This mode focuses on continuous improvement through systematic feedback and reflection. Power is centralised in the system and direction is based on a "vision-mission" that tends to be centrally framed. There is recognition of the importance of distributed knowledge, but this is selective and meaning remains centrally controlled. In this mode the system responds to changes by adapting incrementally. People are viewed as a valuable information resource and individual and group learning is encouraged. Communication is transactional, but more inclusive. This mode relies heavily on rhetorical persuasion, which involves getting people "on board" with a way of thinking. The dominant ideologies are benevolent, yet centralist. Much of Deming's work (explored in Chapter 2) fits with this mode, as does that of his associate Juran. Returning to Juran's Quality Trilogy, this mode maps across to his writings on Quality Improvement. Where the focus is on stabilisation and improvement of processes. Juran makes the important differentiation between firefighting, where changes result in restoration of the previous levels of chronically deficient performance (where the same problem will happen again), and quality improvement, where the changes result in a lasting improvement in performance (Juran, 1989, pp. 28–35).

Mode 3: Relational: "Doing better things" – The emphasis here is on co-production. In this mode change is based on active acknowledgement of multiple stakeholder interests, including the complexity this brings. Power and knowledge are distributed, although not necessarily equally. The mode supports "cross boundary working" especially in situations where multiple interests and stakes prevail and are enduring. People are viewed as resourceful, knowledgeable and competent in

Table 1.1 Three modes of organising (adapted from Anderson-Wallace et al., 2001b, cited in Malby & Anderson-Wallace, 2016)

Mode	Emphasis	Power	Purpose	Knowledge	System Orientation
Mechanistic "Doing things well"	Control	Centralised	Centralised	Centralised	Mechanical
Participative "Doing things better"	Improvement	Centralised	Distributed	Distributed	Whole System/ Complex Adaptive
Relational "Doing better things"	Co-production	Distributed	Distributed	Distributed	Relational/ Complex Responsive

their own situation. Systemic and institutional learning is of particular interest and communication is seen as highly interactive and based on dialogical principles. Following the theme of Juran's trilogy there are some parallels, but also some differences in this mode. Juran emphasised the importance of ensuring that the needs of customers were met, as well as the participation of those most affected (Juran, 1989), but whether he envisaged the level of epistemic inclusion or knowledge equity that are embedded in contemporary notions of co-production is a matter for some debate. Our observation would be that this heavily dialogical approach is rarely seen in quality improvement work, where the purpose of the work is often centrally determined, and the problem already "diagnosed". Other stakeholders may have a role in co-designing the solutions, but this fits better within a Mode 2 approach (Juran, 1989).

As previously mentioned, our belief is that the third mode is of value in addressing complex challenges that cannot be "solved" in a traditional sense, but it is important to re-emphasise that no one mode is inherently "better" than another, and a great deal of collective skill and contextual judgement is needed to decide which approach to adopt in each situation.

What Constitutes Evidence in This Book?

As discussed later in this book, scientific approaches to organisational and management practice claim to have significantly shaped organisational and management practice for more than 150 years, informed by logic, rationality and predictability. For the last 40 years or so, the scientific approach of using randomised controlled trials (RCTs) has been accepted as the "gold standard" of evidence for evaluating new treatments in medicine. The Cochrane Library now contains hundreds of thousands of systematic reviews that follow a predefined protocol to create a standardised method of making sense of vast amounts of clinical research and information (Neuhauser & Diaz, 2007).

It is therefore not surprising that when people working in healthcare – managers and clinicians – ask for "the evidence", they are often referring to something that has been proved using scientific methods. As noted by Neuhauser and Diaz (2007), the fundamental building block of science is generalisable theory, which generates hypotheses that can be put to the test repeatedly through experiments. Simply put, scientific theory makes reality simpler by identifying what is relevant and what is not, what must be controlled for, and allowing us to confidently generalise to different situations. Although quality improvement efforts heavily emphasise the use of statistical data and feedback loops, they have frequently been criticised for not adhering to the same scientific method because their approach is more iterative and less generalisable. This could at least partially explain why the "pilot, spread, and adopt" methods that are so popular in healthcare are often unable to produce the desired results. Put simply, the complexity of the problems people are trying to "solve" are 1) not amenable to this type and "lift and shift" approach and 2) are not in fact solvable in a traditional, scientifically rational sense. We would argue that such methods rarely consider the systemic conditions – the unofficial and official technical, socio-cultural and political influences on the work – that enable a pilot to work, instead tending to focus on the visible tools or method. As Dixon-Woods et al. (2011) point out, a wealth of research demonstrates that trusted peers in addition to formal bodies of evidence and abstract knowledge have an impact on clinical behaviours (Dopson et al., 2003). Therefore, it is crucial to have leaders who can "breathe legitimacy" (Hwang & Powell, 2005) into the ideas being promoted. This is consistent with the more general observation that people are more likely to alter their behaviour when they observe their liked and trusted peers doing the same (Dube & Wilson, 1996). The moral authority of those seeking to use the evidence, as well as the moral communities where those behaviours are practised, must support the evidence's authority for it to be effective. As Wears and Sutcliffe (2019) argue, the combination of the rationality of management and the scientific focus of medicine has created an approach to quality and safety in healthcare that has been significantly self-limiting.

In line with our own inter-disciplinary interests, in this book we take a broad view of what constitutes evidence, drawing on the epistemological, phenomenological, philosophical and empirical. Indeed, given the widely accepted definition of quality explained above – clinical effectiveness, personalisation and safety – it becomes clear quickly that these dimensions do not lend themselves easily to hard-edged scientific method. That said, some elements of the book deeply examine some technical themes, especially when considering issues of variation, demand, capacity and utilisation. This is not because we see these ideas as absolute reflections of truth about the world, but that they provide a language to contextualise and explain. We recognise that some readers will be drawn to different vocabularies and repertories expressed in this book, and others will find them contradictory. All that we ask is that you keep an open mind and consider their "value-in-use" and collectively.

This book certainly does not claim to provide definitive answers, but it does hope to provide some plausible and more effective responses to these complex dilemmas using the lens of "quality". Our evidence – that is to say the account we give for our propositions – takes many forms including studies, opinions, ideas, stories, examples and heuristic frameworks, all of which are offered as approaches to consider problems. Instead of looking for a perfect solution, or the fallacy of a quick win, we encourage you to think about producing pragmatic responses that fall within an acceptable range of accuracy within a reasonable time frame. Our aim is to stimulate thought, conversation and inquiry that enable the next set of actions and meanings to be critically appraised and reflected upon.

What the Book Explores

In chapters 1 to 5, we explore the context of quality thinking and quality improvement (QI) in healthcare. Drawing on the literature, we outline the "his-story" of quality (for it is white Western men who appear to have significantly shaped the narrative thus far) using several key examples to trace the evolution of some of the central ideas. We also explore the often-forgotten conceptual roots of quality, which we refer to in the holistic sense to include experience, effectiveness, efficiency and safety – such as variation, standardisation and utilisation – and consider from industrial and modern management to healthcare – and what to watch out for in their translation. We also consider key questions about demand and capacity – and examine how we can ever know how much work there is to be done, or how much resource is needed to do it and the impact of our often-reactive approach to both in the planning and management of services. We explore in detail the concept of variation – a contested notion – which lies at the heart of much quality thinking and provides us with some method we can use to begin to question our work with curiosity. We also explore the significant, ongoing tension between standardisation and personalisation; autonomy and conformity. These are critical conversations in the healthcare context partly because of the way they invite a move away from the low predictability craft-based approaches – common in traditional medical practice – towards a more predictable, standardised professional approach, which is advocated in more contemporary practice (Boaden, 2009).

We consider the notion of "cultures of quality" including the ways in which norms of practice are formed and reformed in the highly regulated, political space that is the NHS. We will consider what has been learnt about improvements in quality; specifically, the ways in which ideas from sociology and psychology have shaped understanding. We also consider the contributions that quality improvement thinking has made over the past 30 years in health-care, and broadly speaking what research has taught us about the conditions for successful intervention.

In chapters 6 and 7 of the book, we set out a pragmatic framework to improve the analysis of quality problems in healthcare, using the concept of identifying the sources of "Failure Demand" (Seddon, 2008) to inform. This approach considers the immense demands placed on services, which are demands generated by how services are organised and managed, often significantly influenced by complexi-ties in the wider systemic context. We will consider some approaches to reducing Failure Demand, including the traditional hypothesis that the route to quality can be understood through a relentless focus on what "adds value" to the end users in context. We also consider the implications for service design and delivery; for pro-fessional relationships; and for citizen leadership and public participation.

In chapters 8 to 11 we offer four interconnected conceptual domains that we propose as a valuable framework to consider reducing Failure Demand. The frame-work leans heavily on the question of whether we are even doing the right work to begin with; it invites us to focus on the importance of understanding need, including a rethink of the traditional power dynamic between superordinates and subordinates; between specialists and generalists; those who give and receive ser-vices, with a move towards more equity of knowledge within the relationships. We also consider the pressures that can make the workplace a difficult and sometimes damaging place, and advocate some strategies for supporting the human system to include both those who give and receive care.

Some Things to Consider

As you work through this book there are some important principles to hold in mind. These are issues that we as authors have struggled with throughout, and therefore suspect you as the reader might also find a challenge.

Firstly, holding the complexity of the issues that we are discussing has been difficult. It is all too compelling to present issues as binary and abstract – as either this or that; right or wrong; old or new; and so on. The traditional 4x4 matrix or the comparative illustrative tables that we are all so fond of emphasise this, but by doing this we risk falling straight into the modernist trap of atomisation and fragmentation that we are inviting you to critique. And yet, binaries and the sim-plification that they bring can help us to temporarily grasp an idea or a concept to explore it further – in the form of a useful heuristic. So, where we have done this in the book – and we certainly have – our purpose is pragmatic, and our aim is to make the concept more accessible. Any binaries or simplifications are therefore offered "as if" true, rather than "as" true. In practice, the issues remain complex and irreducible. And this brings us to the most challenging aspect of the approach. The ideas we offer are often characterised by paradox (apparent contradictions that co-exist), rather than dualistic certainty (things being either "this or that"). We invite you to "live with" the paradox as it is surely a part of the conditions of uncertainty, fragmentation and complexity that characterise our daily experiences. It is this living with uncertainty, this living with complexity and building of systems that can "hold" both and still deliver on quality, that is the work of leadership in healthcare.

Secondly, this book is not a "how-to" guide, and we unashamedly explore some issues using theoretical frames. Kurt Lewin, the pioneering organisational psychologist, famously noted that there is "nothing as practical as a good theory", and we tend to agree. Lewin considered theories to be merely sets of ideas that describe how something functions. As a result, the practical application of a sound theory is regarded as being of immeasurable value because it allows for the testing of the explanation's logic and the localisation of its practical applications. Additionally, theory enables us to ground our work in data and evidence, both qualitatively and quantitatively, enabling us to explore further. Its purpose is to pique our interest in further research and reflection on current issues, not to offer conclusive solutions.

Finally, we as authors use slightly different vocabularies when we explain things. This difference arises in part because of our respective backgrounds and training in industrial engineering and the psychology of social systems. As you read this book therefore you will notice that in some sections there is an emphasis on the technical aspects of quality – specifically as we explore variation, issues of utilisation, demand and capacity, and so on. In these sections the language tends to be more rational and at times makes more linear causal links – if you like promoting an approach which is akin to "process engineering". In other parts of the book, you will notice a focus on what might be described as "process sociology", where the social nature of organising is strongly in the foreground. In this mode connections are more tangential, and causality is replaced by emergence, uncertainty and complexity. In many ways these differences illustrate the different versions of the notion of systems that are at play in this domain – although they often go unexplored. It is a key area for consideration as healthcare talks more about integration and system-wide working. Our position is that this blending of methods and understandings takes us to a richer and more effective place in terms of questioning and thus improving quality. Our observation of the NHS is that it is rare for the technical and the psychology of human systems to co-exist in any useful depth – usually it is one or the other. This book goes some way to addressing this, suggesting a framework for improving quality for the specific context of healthcare that is firmly rooted in both.

Of course, our vocabularies are the product of the ideologies underpinning the core material, but we hope that neither dominates or makes absolute claims on the truth, and that they add to the plurality of book – reflecting the world within which we live. In summary, and to paraphrase the famous aphorism of British statistician

George Box (1976), we believe that "all models are wrong, but some are useful" – including our own.

We hope that the picture we paint is a refreshing one, and that we can convey the sense of value and confidence we have in these ideas. Our thinking comes from a place of deep reflection, understanding and expertise, but at the same time we also acknowledge it will not be a neat or complete solution. As a minimum, we hope that the book might provide a form of "compass and map" to navigate a world of uncertainty and complexity, but to paraphrase Alfred Korzybski, the 20th-century scientist and philosopher, it is important to remember that "the map is not the territory".

Notes

1 Potage is a thick soup that's usually pureed and is made from whatever vegetables are available. It has its origins in France and was a staple of medieval cuisine.
2 The Griffiths report put an end to consensus management and raised the power and salaries of general managers while reducing the power of other groups. Opposition came from those groups that would lose power, such as public health doctors and nursing managers.
3 Edwards Deming, Joseph Juran and Philip Crosby are widely credited to be influential in the quality thinking we see in today's leaders of quality in healthcare, such as Don Berwick and Brent James – see Chapter 2.

References

Anderson-Wallace, M., Blantern, C., Lejk, A., Gössling, T., Genefke, J., Hosking, D.M., Maas, A.J., Bakker, D.J., MacRae, M., Huxham, C., Vanbeselaere, N. and Wierdsma, A.F.M. 2001a. Conceptualization of dynamics and interventions. In T. Taillieu (ed.), *Collaborative Strategies and Multi-organizational Partnerships* (pp. 155–226). Garant Publishers.

Anderson-Wallace, M., Blantern, C. and Boydell, T. 2001b. Advances in cross-boundary practice: Inter-logics as method. *Career Development International*, 6(7): 414–420.

Bate, S.P. 1994. *Strategies for Culture Change*. Butterworth-Heineman.

Berwick, D.M. 2019. Sounding board: Continuous improvement as an ideal in health care. In R. Stewart (ed.), *Management of Health Care* (pp. 183–186). Routledge.

Boaden, R. 2009. Quality improvement: Theory and practice. *British Journal of Healthcare Management*, 15(1): 12–16.

Boaden, R., Harvey, G., Moxham, C. and Proudlove, N. 2008. *Quality Improvement: Theory and Practice in Healthcare*. NHS Institute for Innovation and Improvement.

Box, G.E.P. 1976. Science and statistics. *Journal of the American Statistical Association*, 71(356): 791–799.

Braithwaite, J. 2018. Changing how we think about healthcare improvement. *BMJ*, 361.

Britain, G. and Darzi, A. 2008. *High Quality Care for All: NHS Next Stage Review Final Report*. Stationery Office.

Committee on Quality of Health Care in America (IOM). 2001. *Crossing the Quality Chasm: A New Health System for the 21st Century*. National Academies Press.

Dixon-Woods, M. 2019. How to improve healthcare improvement – an essay by Mary Dixon-Woods. *BMJ*, 367: l5514.

Dixon-Woods, M., Bosk, C.L., Aveling, E.L., Goeschel, C.A. and Pronovost, P.J. 2011. Explaining Michigan: Developing an ex post theory of a quality improvement program. *The Milbank Quarterly*, 89(2): 167–205.

Donabedian, A. 1966. Evaluating the quality of medical care. *Milbank Memorial Fund Quarterly*, 44(3, Part 2): 166–206.

Dopson, S., Locock, L., Ferlie, E. and Fitzgerald, L. 2003. Evidence-based medicine and the implementation gap. *Health: An Interdisciplinary Journal for the Social Study of Health, Illness and Medicine*, 7(3): 311–330.

Dube, N. and Wilson, D. 1996. Peer education programmes among HIV-vulnerable communities in Southern Africa. In B. Williams and C. Campbell (eds), *HIV/AIDS in the South African Mining Industry* (pp. 107–110). Epidemiology Research Unit.

Griffiths, R. 1983. *NHS Management Inquiry*. DHSS.

Harwood, J. 1986. Ludwik Fleck and the sociology of knowledge. *Social Studies of Science*, 16(1): 173–187.

Hwang, H. and Powell, W.W. 2005. Institutions and entrepreneurship. In H. Hwang and W.W. Powell (eds), *Handbook of Entrepreneurship Research* (pp. 179–210). Kluwer.

Juran, J.M. 1989. *Juran on Leadership for Quality – An Executive Handbook*. Free Press.

Malby, B. and Anderson-Wallace, M. 2016. Leading healthcare networks. In *Networks in Healthcare* (pp. 133–156). Emerald Group Publishing Limited.

Neuhauser, D. and Diaz, M. 2007. Quality improvement research: Are randomised trials necessary? *BMJ Quality & Safety*, 16(1): 77–80.

Seddon, J. 2008. *Systems Thinking in the Public Sector*. Triarchy Press.

Wears, R. and Sutcliffe, K. 2019. *Still Not Safe: Patient Safety and the Middle-Managing of American Medicine*. Oxford University Press.

2

The History of Quality in Healthcare

Framing

In this chapter we will look at some of the most significant contributors to the conceptual development of quality thinking in healthcare over the past 150 years, and explore the genesis of the ideas that silently and often invisibly underpin many of the "taken-for-granted" approaches to quality improvement used today. We explore the effects of the "managerial awakening" of the 19th century and consider how scientific management influenced our thinking about quality during the 20th century and beyond. We'll also explore developments to improve clinical quality in the NHS specifically, both historically and in more recent times, and consider what has been learnt about what works - and what does not.

We will give specific attention to the work of Dr W. Edwards Deming, the so-called father of quality improvement. This is not because we wholeheartedly agree with the approaches he promoted, but because of the legacy of his work in healthcare. We'll explore the four dimensions of his "System of Profound Knowledge" - which promoted an appreciation of "the system" and an understanding of variation within systems, and highlighted the critical influence of theories of knowledge and human psychology on achieving quality - and consider its relevance in a contemporary context (Deming, 2018b).

We explore how "quality thinking" has been used and evolved in healthcare, both in Europe and North America, and introduce several key examples that have shaped the discourse. We have chosen these examples specifically because of the way they point towards a more socio-culturally informed approach to quality and offer an antidote to the proliferation of "tools and techniques" and "quick-fixes" that we feel have come to charac-terise a great deal of quality improvement in healthcare.

As with any historical account, many stories could be told about the influence and rela-tionship between various notable events and characters. We recognise that ours - whilst based on the literature - is simply one of many, and in line with the central thesis of this book, we ask you as the reader to question what has been written and ask what other stories might be told about the relationships between things.

Taylorism and the Legacy of Scientific Management

Although other points could have been chosen to begin our story of quality – for example the Guilds of the 13th century are often cited as early merchant approaches to quality in commerce (Bosshardt & Lopus, 2013) – we have decided to focus on the mid-19th century as a starting point for our account. The Industrial Revolution caused rapid social, economic and technological changes, which in turn led to a seismic shift in how people lived and worked. It was a time of great upheaval. It was also the era of the "managerial awakening", as the ideologies, tools and methods that continue to shape modern managerial discourse emerged quickly.

Frederick W. Taylor, known as the "Father of Modern Management", was devel-oping and promoting a new "scientific method" of management at this time. Taylor's early work concentrated on how work was organised and how efficiency could be increased using the scientific method. His strategy was based on careful observation of production processes, dissecting them into their component parts to the smallest extent possible, and then determining the precise skills needed to achieve peak performance at each stage of the production process. From there, he created standardised techniques that had to be strictly adhered to, thereby produc-ing the desired result at the desired volume. Corresponding measurement systems and financial rewards and penalties were designed to achieve the same goal. A criti-cal dimension was to set the rules for task performance, and to ensure that they were strictly adhered to, and thus an early managerial identity began to emerge (Anderson-Wallace, 2017).

Taylor believed that his early experiments taught him an important lesson: if left to their own devices, individual workers could not, in his view, work out the most efficient way to complete a task and would instead do things the way they had always been done. Taylor therefore argued for a distinct separation between management and employees in terms of decision-making. The manager's job was to fully understand the worker's task before coming up with the best way to com-plete it using scientific methods. Using careful measurement and policing manag-ers would ensure the method was applied correctly, reliably and continuously. You can see the impact of Taylor's influence at all levels of the NHS. Junior and middle ranking staff often have to ask more senior staff to make decisions. Those in commissioning roles often specify the way front line staff should work – and what they should work on. Staff are scrutinised in their work – in fact mechanisms of scrutiny are at an industrial scale in the NHS – with multiple layers. Measurement systems, often with a heavy focus on activity, prevail.

Associates of Taylor, Frank and Lilian Gilbreth (1912) – who jointly developed the time and motion study, which 85 years later formed a central tenet of the NHS's national Productive Series of quality improvement programmes that we explore later in this chapter – and Henry Gantt, who created the planning chart that bears his name and is still widely used today, collaborated with Taylor on many projects. James O. McKinsey, the founder of McKinsey Management Engineers, the predecessor to the still enormously influential Global Management Consultants McKinsey and Co. was another close collaborator. Taylor's work is widely recognised as the world's first universal theory of management and was published as "Principles of Scientific Management" in 1911 (Taylor, 2004). From these collaborations the fundamental tenets of contemporary management were formed (Gantt & Taylor, 2007; Gilbreth, 1912; Fayol, 1916). Illustrating further how well established this early thinking on managerial science is within healthcare today, McKinsey and Company, and other management consultancies, continue to be highly influential in shaping NHS thinking today – with the spend on such management consultancies in the NHS being in the multiple millions every year.

In Europe, Henri Fayol, a French mining engineer, identified a set of five universal management functions in 1916. These still seem remarkably modern in many ways.

Fayol's five functions of management:

1. To forecast and plan: "examining the future and drawing up the plan of action".
2. To organise: "building up the structure, material and human, of the undertaking".
3. To command: "maintaining activity among the personnel".
4. To coordinate: "binding together, unifying and harmonizing all activity and effort".
5. To control: "seeing that everything occurs in conformity with established rule and expressed command".

(Edited from Pugh et al., 1971, cited in Anderson-Wallace, 2017)

The move towards explicit, standardised methods and rules based on this "science" was seen as both revolutionary and highly efficient in terms of productivity and financial performance. Many applauded the move away from the previously "highly personalized, idiosyncratic, and unpredictable behaviours of business owners, and often repressive autocracies that preceded them" (Anderson-Wallace, 2017 p. 171).

This move though, it should be noted, is not uniform in the NHS. While some routes to leadership are highly professionalised, such as the NHS Management Training Scheme, some feature tiny amounts of training, development and support in comparison – typically as clinicians take up leadership positions. This opens up the risk of idiosyncrasy and unpredictability in leadership as described by Pugh et al. 2001 in their writings on Fayol.

These early theories and methods continued to serve as the ideological foundation for many Western organisations during the 20th century, even though the language of management may have changed. Generations of management practitioners and academics have been influenced by the discourses and narratives that these largely uncontested aspects of contemporary management practice have produced.

Through the influence of the increasingly potent and intricately intertwined business schools and management consultancies, our understandings of mainstream organisational design, structure and managerial identity were subtly shaped, strengthened and reinforced (Micklethwaite & Wooldridge, 1996). As Morgan (1996) points out, the "organisation in our heads" is still largely based on the principles of classical management theory including the apparent certainties that lie in their social structures.

The Emergence of Quality Thinking

Early in the 20th century, technological and social change continued to occur quickly. One such change was the widespread adoption of mass production, which depended on standardised procedures running continuously to produce outputs of consistent quality.

We first notice the emergence of quality thinking in this setting. W. Edwards Deming, often referred to as the "father of quality improvement", played a significant role in this story. Throughout his writings and his practice, on the quality problems of production at this new unprecedented scale, Deming's central thesis revolved around three main conceptual themes which included the importance of people; the value of co-operation; and the deadliness of wasted resources (Deming, 2018a).

Deming's early formative experiences of organisational life began during the summers of 1924 and 1925 when he worked at Western Electrics, a company at the forefront of the technical revolution in the mass production of telephone equipment. The plant was already engaged in a great deal of innovative practice and made famous by the so-called "Hawthorne experiments" on industrial productivity, led by social psychologist Elton Mayo and colleagues (Mayo, 1933). These experiments were numerous and wide ranging, but in summary claimed to show how changes in the work environment – from hours of work to rest, boredom, fatigue, incentives, and even lighting – all affected human performance. Although Deming was not directly involved with these experiments, the conclusions resonated strongly with his emerging ideas about the inter-relatedness of work problems and strengthened his views about the importance of focusing on the conditions of employees.

Deming was fascinated by the human dimension of work and curious about how the "system conditions" – as they became known – shaped human behaviour. He was especially keen to move away from focusing on problems relating to the failings of individuals, preferring to understand this as being related to the system. He famously introduced the 94/6 rule – meaning that in his view 94% of all problems were attributable to the interacting, inter-related variables within the system or process, and only 6% to "special cause" (i.e. the individual). This early approach to "systems thinking" also encouraged analysis and consideration of the interaction between people, processes, materials and environments, and invited managers to hold the complexity of these interactions and resist the atomisation of problems. This was in direct conflict with a central feature of the dominant scientific management approach. Although Deming's approach could be seen as "systems" focused, this early understanding of systems still tended to be focused on process flows and was linear in conception. It did, however, acknowledge the influence of multiple variables, the limited influence individuals at certain levels have on their own system of work, and to some extent began to acknowledge some of the messiness of organisational life.

During his time at Western Electric, Deming met his mentor and long-term collaborator, Dr Walter A. Shewhart, a physicist and statistician. Shewhart is most famous for the design and development of a data-driven approach to quality control known as statistical process control or SPC, which is discussed in greater detail in Chapter 4. Deming continued to work with Shewhart after their time at Western Electric, collaborating to develop the now famous "Plan-Do-Study-Act" cycle, also sometimes known by many as the Shewhart Cycle for learning and improvement. This approach interfered with the taken-for-granted models of change, and encouraged an iterative process, based on small tests of change to understand the effects of various interdependencies. The PDSA cycle is still seen as a fundamental part of most QI methodology today (Boaden et al., 2008). Interest in Shewhart's work grew rapidly and was sustained over many years. In the late 1980s when Motorola developed a philosophy for quality improvement, they put Shewhart's ideas at their core. They called this approach "Six Sigma" (Dahlgaard & Mi Dahlgaard-Park, 2006).

But Deming is probably best known for his work helping to rebuild the Japanese industrial base, which had been decimated by the effects of the Second World War. Deming was instrumental in the development of a wide range of integrated socio-technical improvement methods, many of which were said to have contributed to the position of competitive advantage enjoyed by many Japanese companies during the 1980s and 1990s. The most famous of these was the "Toyota Production System" (TPS), which for many years was the gold standard for quality control in manufacturing (Ohno, 2019). The TPS model, codified into the five Lean Principles in the hugely popular book *Lean Thinking* by Dan Jones and James Womack (2003), was adapted for use in a wide range of settings, including healthcare. The Virginia Mason Production System, which incorporates Deming's familiar triple mantra of respect for people; continuous improvement; and the management of waste, has been widely held up as one of the best applied examples of quality improvement in the healthcare context (Nelson-Peterson & Leppa, 2007).

Deming concluded his career with two seminal texts: *Out of Crisis* (Deming, 2018a), which defined his 14 points for management, and *The New Economics* (Deming, 2018b), which was arguably the first philosophy of management grounded in systems theory. Fundamental to *The System of Profound Knowledge* (SPK) explored in the New Economics was the need to understand "work" as a system of inter-related connections, interactions and dependencies as opposed to the then more common, traditional understanding of the work as discreet and independent departments and processes governed by various chains of command. SPK was perhaps one of the first philosophies of management that appreciated the power of context and acknowledged the different risks that are experienced locally within sub-systems as important variables to consider. The approach increased the focus on problems in quality as attributable to "the system" rather than special causes – outwith the system – such as blaming an individual for mistakes.

Deming's view of "the system" could be said to draw on an approach to systems thinking, which understands them as the "whole" formed by the interaction of "parts". Causality is the process by which interactions between the parts take shape. The method also places a strong emphasis on realism, which means that the system is viewed as a mental framework developed between different people or groups of people. Deming was not the only person at the time to develop these concepts; researchers from many disciplines, including biology, psychology, sociology, engineering, and communications, were also working to refine their systems thinking methodologies. These ways of thinking certainly amounted to a new paradigm, although as previously discussed, the mechanistic approach to management and organising was still highly operative in practice. Deming also felt that giving careful attention to "aims" was especially important as in his view this was how systems developed their sense of direction and purpose. He believed very strongly that quality emerged when individuals were "committed or enrolled" – in other words, personally invested in the task. As significantly, he felt that focusing on compliance with organisational rules and regulations created perverse incentives and demanded an approach to management supervision that was based on policing rather than support. He fundamentally believed that linking to intrinsic rather than extrinsic motivations was how quality could be fostered. These features can be seen in many contemporary approaches to quality improvement in healthcare (see examples in Chapter 3 for a more detailed discussion).

Deming was a strong proponent of natural altruism and thought that extrinsic motivations like rewards and punishments were seriously harmful to the advancement of quality.

He believed that the main tenets of Taylorism had imposed excessive restrictions, overly standardised the process, and ultimately demanded excessive conformity. He despised the "carrot and stick" methods of management because he saw them as idolisation and punishment, with shame being a powerful tool for change. He thought that this had the effect of crushing the human spirit and dehumanising the workplace, which eventually produced feelings of demoralisation and alienation.

Deming emphasised the absolute necessity of understanding the human condition to achieve any improvement in quality. He put this in a psychological context. He believed that people are fundamentally social beings who were born in need of respect, love and attachment. He had a positive outlook on what motivated people to act and believed that curiosity, the joy of learning, and achievement were the fundamental components of what it meant to be human.

People are motivated to act altruistically - Joy is derived from this altruism; through intangible feelings and the sense of warmth and satisfaction that arises. If you begin to reward altruism extrinsically - by awards, bonuses and the like - we risk discontinuing the altruistic behaviour. (Deming, 2018b)

The idea of epistemology, or the theories of knowledge, is perhaps one of the most difficult aspects of the System of Profound Knowledge, and arguably the dimension that became obscured as others "cherry-picked" across his ideas. Deming essentially challenged us to reflect on how we come to know what we do and to carefully consider the ideologies, convictions and philosophies that shape how work is perceived, created and provided. He also emphasised the negative consequences of not challenging these presumptions, particularly the harm caused by focusing only on the evidence that confirms our current beliefs and ignoring that which might contradict or refute our theories. This is particularly important in healthcare because many of the philosophies and beliefs are founded in professional and technical belief systems that have their roots in medicine, as well as sometimes unknowingly in the principles of scientific management.

Deming's final text *The New Economics* was completed in the year of his death, and arguably was a more accessible and mainstream exposition of his ideas. In this book he concluded firmly that co-operation rather than competition was the only way to achieve long-term market success via the route of learning, innovation and "deep joy at work". He also identified what were described as the "Seven Deadly Diseases of Management":

---

1. Lack of constancy of purpose
2. Emphasis on short term (profits) results
3. Evaluation of performance, merit ratings or annual reviews
4. Mobility of management - job hopping
5. Management only by use of visible figures with no consideration of the unknowable/unknown
6. Excessive medical costs (costs of employee dis-ease)
7. Excessive costs of liability - amplified by lawyers working on contingency fees

(Deming, 2018b)

Whilst these points may seem obvious on paper, they were revolutionary at the time and remain challenging to the NHS and other healthcare systems to date, particularly because they are a direct challenge to the very dominant mechanistic and reductionist ideologies and practices of Taylorism and scientific management.

There is no doubt that Deming's contribution to the quality movement was enormous. He challenged Taylorism and its mechanical metaphors and language, and expounded an approach which took account of multiple variables and acknowledged the complexity and messiness of human interactions. However, as Stacey and Mowles (2016) point out, although Deming and others were actively contesting the rather negative perspective that Taylor and Fayol took of humans in the workplace, arguing that "the role of the manager was to organise teamwork and so sustain co-operation" (p. 60), they did not abandon the scientific management approach. Instead, they used scientific methods to study group motivation. As they state, "The blend of scientific management and human relations produce a theoretical position that still relied on the idea that organisational stability is preserved by rules – including those influencing motivation – which in turn govern the behaviour of members of an organisation" (p. 59).

According to Stacey and Mowles (2016), even though Deming thought that best performance was attained when people are treated with respect and are motivated – as opposed to being policed thorough standard, protocol-driven work practices and/or penalised financially – the process of improvement is still thought to be facilitated by managers' intervention and how they alter the rules and conditions. This strategy is predicated on the notion that managers can influence system conditions through logical decision-making, which then results in the desired changes in a linear and uncomplicated manner. The fundamental assumption about workers – which is essentially a Taylorist one – remains that they are relatively ignorant and require rules and conditions to be set up for them to perform at their best. Although the shift away from the de-humanising machine metaphors of Taylorism – with people characterised as "cogs in a machine" – was important, the humanists replaced this with a horticultural metaphor. In this analogy the workers are now the seeds within the garden, and managers the benevolent gardeners, creating the conditions for optimal growth using their superior knowledge and skills. The overall aim is still for growth, productivity and maximum efficiency, but this time it is achieved by manipulating the "system conditions" and working on individual motivation. Despite significant critique over many years, Deming's ideas are still hugely influential in management thinking and have reinforced a powerful and potentially patronising relationship between workers and managers.

Total Quality Management, Continuous Quality Improvement and Business Process Re-Engineering

The "Total Quality Management" (TQM) movement, which attracted significant attention in a variety of industrial and commercial settings during the late 1980s and early 1990s, is widely credited with having been launched by Deming's book *Out of Crisis*, even though he never used the term. TQM was somewhat overshadowed by the widespread adoption of the Toyota Production System, the rise of lean manufacturing practices, and the adoption of six sigma methodologies at General Electric under the direction of CEO Jack Welch. When compared to the control group, the research conducted at hundreds of US companies that had won awards for implementing TQM initially showed impressive performance, but the outcomes over time were much more variable (Hendricks & Singhal, 2000, 2001; Stacey & Mowles, 2016).

Despite significant promotion of the approach in the 1990s, Blumenthal and Kilo (1998) noted that they could not identify a healthcare organisation that had fundamentally improved its performance through Continuous Quality Improvement (CQI). There were no empirical studies of TQM or CQI and performance in healthcare organisations. Blumenthal and Scheck (1995) also noted a significant and problematic gap between the language of quality and that of medicine, as well as a great deal of scepticism on the part of medical staff involved in TQM work. Berwick et al. (1991), who had played a significant role in several national demonstration projects for quality improvement in healthcare, concluded that "barriers to physician involvement may turn out to be the most important single issue impeding the success of quality improvement in medical care" (p. 151). Boyne and Walker (2002) came to the same conclusion in their critical review that there was no solid proof of TQM's beneficial effects on performance. Despite this evidence, many managers passionately believed that the quality improvement programmes had been successful. Simply put, there appeared to be a substantial difference between the story that was lived and the evaluation evidence.

The evaluations of TQM and CQI projects showed a consistent pattern of variable impact and most struggled to find reliable methods to measure. The overall conclusion was that quality improvements could only be achieved when the conditions for success – often referred to as the receptive context – were in place. These included sustained leadership focus, adequate support and education, data systems and measurement that were reliable, and importantly protection from overburdensome regulation (Shortell et al., 1998). In the UK, it was also noted that the conditions for successful implementation were generally absent. On the whole projects were seen to be fragmented and appeared to rely on a small number of highly competent and committed individuals who supported their design and implementation.

Business Process Re-Engineering (BPR), which gained significant traction in the early 1990s, was another related strategy for enacting radical organisational change. Aiming to move away from disconnected task performance and restructure to create more effective processes, BPR sought to map and analyse workflow both within and across functions. The horizontal process structures that were used in place of hierarchical functional structures were said to be a rejection of the mechanistic industrial paradigm by the invention's creators. BPR placed a strong emphasis on the concepts of self-management and empowerment within core processes, and those who took part in the process were seen as having the most to offer in the way of improvements since they were the process experts themselves. Furthermore, it was thought that the self-managed team framework allowed quick decisions to be made and actions to be taken without interrupting crucial workflows (Anderson-Wallace, 2017).

In the mid- to late 1990s, at both Kings Healthcare, London and Leicester Royal Infirmary, a large-scale application of BPR was made in the context of UK healthcare (Bowns & McNulty, 1999; McNulty & Ferlie, 2004). The project's goals were extremely ambitious, but despite an initial strong adherence to the traditional BPR method, this eventually gave way to a more gradual and continuous approach to redesign. Although there were some obvious advantages in terms of service redesign and financial savings, quantitative data suggested that the impact was much less significant than projected in the business case. Briefly stated, the formal evaluation contends that the project was evolutionary as opposed to revolutionary, with some incremental improvement as opposed to the radical transformation that was promised. While there were some significant and sustained service improvements, the overall effect of individual projects on patient care was inconsistent. These initiatives seemed to show that BPR's potential for bringing about fundamental organisational change in the public sector was, at best, unproven (Anderson-Wallace, 2017; Bowns & McNulty, 1999; McNulty & Ferlie, 2004).

Improving Clinical Quality

One could argue that methods for enhancing clinical quality, or more precisely methods for enhancing efficiency and results in healthcare, are as old as the medical professions themselves. Boaden et al. (2008) link the history of clinical quality improvement with the conceptualisation of clinical work as a craft, which many associate with the so-called founding father of medicine Sir William Osler in the late 19th century. We begin this part of our story around a similar time but with the Hungarian physician and scientist, Ignaz Semmelweis, who pioneered work to understand anti-septic techniques. His proposal was met with strong opposition despite compelling evidence that hand washing with chlorinated lime solutions had a critical role to play in reducing puerperal fever, a bacterial infection that frequently killed new mothers soon after giving birth. Semmelweis meticulously gathered and presented his data, recording the occurrence and frequency of infections over time, as well as the sharp decline that occurred when anti-septic techniques were applied. The suggestion that they wash their hands, though, deeply offended his co-workers, who relentlessly mocked him for it. As he became increasingly outspoken in his views and despite convincing evidence from his data, he was ostracised. A little over four years after finishing his ground-breaking work, Semmelweis was committed to an asylum, where he later died following an alleged attack by asylum guards.

Many years after his death, Louis Pasteur confirmed his theories, and Joseph Lister, the French microbiologist, successfully proved hygienic and anti-septic methods. Only then was his work fully recognised. Anyone who has tried to improve quality in a healthcare environment is likely to at least partially recognise the pattern of response that Semmelweis encountered (stopping short of being beaten to death we hope). However, in all seriousness, as Aveling et al. (2012) note, gaining collegiate support from within the clinical community is of the utmost importance in creating any improvement. We will discuss this in greater detail in Chapter 3.

Florence Nightingale, the English nurse, was another data-driven "quality improver" in the 19th century. Nightingale, known as "the lady with the lamp", might be as appropriately referred to as "the lady with the pie chart". In the military field hospital she oversaw, Nightingale's "rose diagram", which is comparable to the modern histogram, was used to show the seasonal causes of patient mortality. Although she did not develop the technique, she was a pioneer in the use of infographics and data visualisation during the Crimean War. She persisted in using statistical analyses to shape social policy at the highest levels, and in 1859, she was elected as the Royal Statistical Society's first female member (Aravind & Chung, 2010; Strachey, 2013). In common with other successful quality improvers in healthcare whose stories we touch on in this chapter, Semelweiss and Nightingale used data-driven approaches to both understand the nature of the problem and the impact of their interventions. Perhaps most significantly however, they attempted to intervene – knowingly and not knowingly – at a cultural level within their clinical communities, disrupting the dominant discourse within their respective professional domains.

An early version of clinical audit was created in 1916 by US surgeon Ernest Codman as he began to concentrate on the process of evaluating the outcomes of medical interventions.

Avedis Donabedian went a step further and created a multi-dimensional concept of quality in the 1960s and 1970s. Donabedian was not only concerned with the technical quality of care; he was also interested in the social context in which it was provided and the doctor–patient relationship (Donabedian, 1966). His now-famous "structure-process-outcome" model encouraged a significantly more systemic way of thinking about medical care, and consequently quality. He was renowned for emphasising the moral and ethical aspects of care, as succinctly stated in the quotation:

Systems awareness and systems design are important for health professionals, but they are not enough. They are enabling mechanisms only. It is the ethical dimensions of individuals that are essential to a system's success. Ultimately, the secret of quality is love.

By the 1980s, Donald Berwick, a Harvard-trained paediatrician who developed an interest in "Quality-of-Care Measurement" while working at the Harvard Community Health Plan, had begun to test the viability of applying industrial models of quality improvement. He drew heavily on the quality gurus Deming, Juran and Shewhart (discussed earlier in this chapter) and was certain that quality control mechanisms could be useful in the healthcare context. Berwick was, and continues to be, a strong follower of Deming's philosophies, describing his early experience of attending one of Deming's famous four-day courses as an "emotionally challenging and life changing experience" during which he realised that his "well-intentioned attempts to improve quality through inspection and correction were counter-productive and led to an erosion of 'pride-in-work'" (Berwick, 2016).

Crossing the Quality Chasm

Remarkably, given the significant work on quality and systems in other contexts during the early part of the 20th century, it wasn't until 1999 that the Institute of Medicine (IoM) in the US published a seminal report that first defined what "quality" meant in a healthcare context.

The IoM report was motivated by a growing realisation that fundamental reform of the US healthcare system was needed to address the population's profound changes in knowledge, technology and health needs, not to mention the rising cost of healthcare.

It was obvious that the severely disjointed delivery system, which lacked even the most basic clinical information capability, was causing duplication, protracted wait times and delays. Most alarmingly, the report found that neither quality nor cost issues within the healthcare system were addressed, nor was it made clear that waste was pervasive.

In essence, it concluded that the current healthcare system was ineffective. The report made a persuasive case for adopting quality as a system of property, supported by high-quality information technology to support clinical and administrative processes, as well as a more collaborative leadership style that could function across organisational boundaries (Baker, 2001).

Six key aims for improvements were identified:

---

1. *Safe care* – to avoid injuries from the care that is intended to help patients
2. *Effective care* – based on the best scientific knowledge, avoiding under or overuse respectively
3. *Patient-centred care* – which was respectful and responsive to individual patient preferences, needs and values
4. *Timely care* – which reduced waiting and harmful delays
5. *Efficient care* – that avoided waste of equipment, supplies, energy and ideas
6. *Equitable care* – which did not vary in quality based on personal characteristics such as gender, ethnicity, location or socio-economic status

(Adapted from Baker, 2001)

The IoM report was undoubtedly a bold, reasoned and persuasive call to action, with specific suggestions for how the six objectives might be best achieved. Its conclusions were remarkably obvious on one level. With the patient as the source of control, strong proposals for new rules to redesign and improve care were made, including moving care towards continuous healing relationships based on needs and values. It promoted a method of knowledge exchange and open communication between doctors and patients, highlighting the significance of openness and honesty. It put the use of evidence when making decisions at the centre of this information exchange. With the intention of preventing and mitigating error through greater attention to systemic conditions, safety of care was positioned as a key system property. Strongly recommended was a more proactive approach to understanding patient needs coupled with a clear focus on reducing resource waste, with the time of both patients and clinicians firmly incorporated into this equation. Finally, the report made the case for improved clinician collaboration in support of improved care coordination and integration. The report acknowledged the size of the task at hand and the necessary adjustments for a notable improvement in the country's healthcare system. Additionally, it is suggested that payment policies be in line with quality enhancements related to the six aims. The report was a potent intervention that received strong backing from the medical field. Most importantly, it sparked a variety of important discussions about healthcare quality in the USA and the UK.

By the turn of the 21st century, definitions of clinical quality were appearing quickly. In 2003, John Øvretveit's defined quality improvement in the healthcare context as "better patient experience and outcomes achieved through changing provider behaviour and organisation through using a systematic change method and strategies" (Øvretveit & Gustafson, 2003).

New Labour, Modernisation and the Breakthrough Series Collaboratives

After 18 years of Conservative rule, Tony Blair's New Labour won a resounding victory in 1997, signalling the beginning of a new era for the NHS. A new long-term modernisation plan was created with the goal of saving the NHS, which was part of the New Labour platform. The NHS Plan, which was published in 2000, was supported by a pledge to increase NHS funding from 4.5% to 9% of GDP, in line with that of European counterparts. With this enormous infusion of new funding into the system came great demands for reform, including ambitious targets in priority areas such as specific disease areas of cancer and coronary heart disease; commitments on access; and long-overdue goals to reduce iatrogenic harm, particularly healthcare-associated infections like MRSA.

It was understood that a supporting infrastructure would be needed to speed up the changes required, and the NHS Modernization Agency (MA) was established. The organisation was soon rapidly expanded, based on "a sufficiently strong impression on Government" from the early programmatic approaches to service and quality improvement (Ham et al., 2002, p. 12). The MA was the first in a line of national organisations devoted to enhancing quality and services in the NHS, starting a ten-year process of extensive improvement initiatives.

A substantial part of the work was framed by the Institute for Healthcare Improvement (IHI) Model for Improvement based on Deming's work, and the Breakthrough Series Collaborative (BTS), which was created in response to the many TQM and CQI pilots of the 1990s, was chosen as the main methodology (McLeod & Peck, 2005). Over the course of the following 12 years Professor Don Berwick, who was the IHI's President at the time, served as an advisor to the Modernisation Agency and the national improvement agencies that followed. Berwick received an Honorary Knighthood for his work in UK healthcare in 2005, underlining his contribution to the quality movement in healthcare.

The IHI's BTS methodology incorporated many of Deming's well-known themes, such as a focus on empowering those who are closest to the work, carefully defined evidence-based topics with specific aims and a clear gap between current state and best practice, a supportive and collaborative inter-organisational infrastructure, and a short timeframe for activity in which ambitious dramatic changes were imagined.

Key principles of BTS collaborative model:

- A bottom-up approach in which activities are changed incrementally to create new processes which generate high-quality outcomes
- A focus on a carefully defined topic in which there is a clear gap between current and best practice
- Networking across organisations to shorten the time for identifying aims, diagnoses and remedies
- A package of support to facilitate networking, CQI skills development, topic-related evidence base and a structured implementation model
- A short timeframe in which ambitious and dramatic change is expected

(Adapted from Kilo, 1998)

The strategy was based on 47 collaboratives that were conducted in the US between 1995 and 2003, ten of which saw "breakthrough" successes reported by the teams. A "breakthrough" was defined as a 20% to 40% improvement over predetermined metrics; 7 out of 12 participants in the later collaboratives (58%) reported "breakthroughs".

Physician engagement was noted as a major issue for the US collaboratives, and it was noted that one of the most frequent reasons for failure early in the process was an extended preoccupation with data collection, which was motivated by the conventional view that "proof" of the severity of the issue was required before any attempt could be made to change the process (Leape et al., 1998).

The effectiveness of the approach in comparison to other organisational development interventions is still debatable, despite careful consideration being given to the conditions that appear to be important in setting up and managing these large-scale temporary learning systems by those independently evaluating a range of BTS collaboratives in a number of countries (Mittman, 2004; Øvretveit et al., 2002). There is a great deal of discussion here about whether the methodology is flawed or whether the participating organisations' prevailing cultural conditions are what prevent long-term implementation. Similar to TQM/CQI, participants' qualitative feedback in many of the large-scale collaboratives seems to support their value, particularly in fostering social capital and knowledge. However, whether the BTS methodology produces better results than other forms of social learning and knowledge management approaches seems debatable. Mittman (2004) emphasises that:

> the widespread acceptance and reliance on this approach are based not on solid evidence but on shared beliefs and anecdotal affirmations that may overstate the actual effectiveness of the method. More effective use of the collaborative method will require a commitment by users, researchers, and other stakeholders to rigorous, objective evaluation and the creation of a valid, useful knowledge and evidence base. (Mittman, 2004, p. 897)

Although no conclusive evidence was found, researchers hypothesised that a team's success or failure depended on five broad factors. These included their capacity for teamwork, their aptitude for using quality techniques, the strategic significance of their work to their home organisations, the culture of those organisations, and the kind and level of management support (Mittman, 2004).

Based on personal experience, we would note that the overstating of results continues to be a common theme. This may have to do with the optimism bias that afflicts many worthy and important initiatives in healthcare. Put simply, to secure resources and time in a highly utilitarian system, people and departments must wildly overstate the likely outcomes of their work, often promising to resolve intractable problems over impossible timescales to secure commitment. If they didn't do this, against a backdrop of effective internal competition for resources they would not be heard. The consequence for organisations is this raises the odds that the "projects chosen for funding and resource will have the highest probability for disappointment" (Lovallo & Kahnerman, 2003).

McLeod (2005) argued that the success of the BTS collaboratives was largely determined by professionals, particularly doctors. Citing Mintzberg (1979), he makes the case that if we think of healthcare as a type of professional bureaucracy, where groups of people collaborate to access shared resources and assistance but otherwise function largely independently, then their commitment to a more integrated approach may be in doubt. Change and improvement are viewed in this context less as a co-operative effort and more as a series of negotiations that involve "partisan mutual adjustments" (Pettigrew et al., 1992, p. 14). There seems to be a direct conflict here, which does not sit well with the development of a temporary multi-organisational learning system.

Despite ongoing debates about efficacy, the IHI Breakthrough Series Collaborative methodology was adopted as a primary method for advancing quality in healthcare in the NHS during the 2000s. The approach has also been adopted to support a wide range of initiatives for over 20 years and has spawned various quality improvement networks including the regional Advancing Quality Alliance, NHS Quest (a member-led QI network) and the Health Foundation Q Initiative, who adapted and used a range of QI approaches to support learning and development at scale.

"High Quality Care for All"

In 2008, "High Quality Care for All" (Britain & Darzi, 2008) was published as a Government White Paper. It defined clinical quality in the NHS for the first time and building on the IoM report identified the triumvirate of safety, patient-centeredness and clinical effectiveness as the key dimensions of quality. Quality was proposed as the organising principle of the NHS and the reforms were widely welcomed. *The Lancet* triumphantly announced that:

Darzi has wisely thrown out regulation as the organising principle of the NHS. He has replaced it with quality... This cultural shift is a radical revisioning of purpose for the NHS - away from the political command and control processes and towards professional responsibility for clinical outcomes. (Horton, 2008)

Around the same time Professor Don Berwick shared a list of principles as a 60th birthday gift to NHS in England. These were firmly based on Deming's work.

Berwick's advice to the NHS on its 60th birthday.

1. Put the patient at the absolute centre of your system of care
2. Stop restructuring
3. Strengthen the local healthcare systems
4. Reinvest in general practice and primary care
5. Don't put your faith in market forces
6. Avoid supply driven care like the plague
7. Develop an integrated approach to assessment, assurance and improvement of quality
8. Heal the divide between the professionals, managers and government
9. Train your healthcare workforce for the future not the past
10. Aim for health

(Berwick, 2008)

Meanwhile in the US, building on the IoM report, Berwick was developing what became known as the Triple Aim for Healthcare, an approach to improving quality in a system by looking at three key areas: population health, the experience of care – including safety, clinical effectiveness and so on – and the reduction of per capita cost, including looking at waste elimination and reducing of cost. The resonance from Deming's early work is easily recognisable in this work, although the emphasis on supporting people is perhaps a little more opaque.

It is interesting to note that despite Berwick repeating his advice to the highest levels of the NHS and Government over more than two decades, including a detailed report in response to the Public Inquiry looking at the care failings at Mid Staffordshire NHS Foundation Trust, the system of regulation and inspection in the NHS continues to be the primary method of managing quality at a system level to this day. This position was arguably strengthened by the establishment and development of the Care Quality Commission (CQC) in 2009, shortly after the publication of "High Quality Care for All", which sets quality standards for individual organisations – not systems of care – against which they are inspected and regulated. The CQC system of regulation and inspection was developed following the Francis Inquiry, and now is about to take on added responsibilities for inspecting Integrated Care Boards, the new collaborative forms of governance introduced as part of the 2022 Health and Care Act.

The Productive Series

Drawing heavily from the thinking and tools of Lean, the Productive Series of national QI programmes were a series of setting-specific initiatives designed to spread quality improvement and improve productivity at scale within the NHS. Developed between 2007 and 2016 by the NHS Institute for Innovation and Improvement, the successor organisation to the NHS Modernization Agency, they achieved the spread of QI techniques at a scale never achieved previously, with adoption reported by 80% of English NHS Trusts (Williams et al., 2019) and 70% of all English NHS acute wards reporting implementing the Productive Ward (NHS Institute for Innovation and Improvement, cited in Sarre et al., 2020). Crucially this was done without central mandate. The ward-based series of QI activities initially used the strapline "Releasing Time to Care" which was considered to resonate with the motivations of patient-facing staff working at the sharp end of delivery. It is interesting to note, however, that the programme soon lost the strapline and became known by all as simply "The Productive Ward", emphasising the focus on productivity rather than care. QI programmes within the series included ward-based approaches in acute and mental health settings, operating theatres, community hospital, community services and general practice. Programmes in the series were licensed internationally and adopted by other health systems. It was whilst contributing to a number of the programmes in this series that we the authors met and began our journey of seeking to understand and improve quality in healthcare – something we have been doing together for 20+ years since.

While the Productive Series was proven to show local benefits for staff and patients and increases in patient contact time (Williams et al., 2019), like previous

QI initiatives much was not sustained systemically with most trusts reporting to survey research in 2018 by Sarre et al. that the Productive Ward was no longer in use. Half of the nursing directors who responded to the surveys reported that the programme had influenced future improvement strategies in their trusts (Sarre et al., 2020). The Productive Series deliberately took the position to focus on the "how not the what" (NHS England Improvement Hub, n.d.). To support the work, rather than question it. The assumption being that the work was broadly right, it just needed optimising, and that front line staff would or could determine if that was the case before seeking to improve it. For example, should this person even be on this ward in the first place? Is this intervention I am trying to improve the efficiency of even effective? Or, as a GP, am I merely treating symptoms or addressing the conditions that are generating this ill-health? Returning to the typology from Anderson-Wallace, Blantern and Boydell's three modes of organising explored in Chapter 1, the assumption was that the staff could differentiate between the need to "do things better" (making incremental improvements to exsiting ways of working) and the need to "do better things" (reframe the nature of the work completely) (2001). In our subsequent work we have observed that busy clinical staff often do not have either the time (headspace), agency or permission to do this. The danger that arose through this approach was that the "wrong" work was simply being made more efficient. Other contributory factors for differing success in different providers was the varying levels of rigor in adoption – especially in providers (by this we mean hospitals adopting the programmes) considering the socio-cultural dimensions of change. It was another assumption that provider management teams would have the capability and understanding to do this.

In many ways, the Productive Series was a triumph of accessibility and spread of simple QI tools, but with variable impact. It showed that it was possible to galvanise tens of thousands of staff to attempt to improve quality without requiring a mandate, at a time before social media. What the series did not do was help or encourage clinicians to question their work in the way we are advocating in this book.

Post 2012

The 2012 Health and Social Care reforms saw the dissolution of the NHS Institute for Innovation and Improvement and the abolition of the National Patient Safety Agency. This ended more than a decade of activity to improve quality at a large scale within the NHS, with responsibility for quality devolving to local and regional commissioning organisations and a much smaller national team that remained a division of the NHS Commissioning Board for England. This brought quality and safety at a national level firmly into the domain of regulation and inspection. The CQC as the independent regulator developed a more extensive system of inspection for all healthcare providers in England. The devolved administrations in

Wales, Scotland and Northern Ireland continued to broadly follow the strategic approaches developed by Don Berwick and colleagues at the Institute for Healthcare Improvement, through a range of formal partnerships. Several larger Foundation Trusts in England did the same, and although these organisations often claimed to continue to improve quality, it is hard to say whether this was as a direct result of the approaches adopted or because of other contextual factors.

However, the 2012 reforms did not signal the end of the story for quality improvement at a national level in England. By 2015, the then Secretary of State for Health, Rt Hon Jeremy Hunt MP, visited the Virginia Mason Institute (VMI) in the US and became interested in the Virginia Mason Production System approach, modelled on the Toyota Production System. He decided to support a five-year partnership to test the model in five participating NHS organisations in England. The partnership's goal was to help each Trust to create a customised version of the Virginia Mason Production System based on "lean" principles. The goal was to establish and support a continuous improvement in capability culture within each of these organisations, from which the wider NHS might learn. The effects of the VMI partnership were investigated by a team of researchers at Warwick Business School.

Early data from 2018–19 identified that three out of the five Trusts had achieved widescale improvements in financial position, quality of care and staff morale. However, two out of the five Trusts had achieved improvements but were within the "special measures" regime of the CQC. Several crucial practices appear to have encouraged continuous improvement. The development of a compact – a non-binding informal agreement on expected conduct and commitments – was thought to allow network governance and inter-organisational learning to take place. The compact provided a safe space for relationships with co-workers and the regulators to ease the negotiation of new norms and roles in a more collaborative way, particularly when they conflicted with established institutional practices or regulatory expectations (Burgess et al., 2019).

The Partnership's final report, which was released in late 2022, states that the project showed that some impressive operational improvements were possible. The five Trusts reduced waste and sped up various processes by a combined 62%, generating considerable time savings every year, with patient services significantly improved, according to the trial's analysis. However, these successes are qualified by a note of caution that the scale of sustained improvement needed in the NHS in England is significant and the report authors argue that the adoption of a systematic and integrated approach that covers entire organisations and systems rather than a patchwork of small interventions dispersed among hospitals would be needed to achieve this (Burgess et al., 2022).

A strong culture of peer learning and knowledge sharing was identified as a critical enabler of organisation-wide improvement. A social network analysis (SNA) showed that the best performing organisations showed a high degree of connectivity between people within a widely distributed network, with dense clusters and grouping indicating high degrees of collaboration across boundaries. Those organisations that fared less well still showed an ability to grasp the technical side of the implementation, but the SNA showed more decentralised, chain-like connections between people, with less density showing low to moderate connectivity and limited engagement and knowledge sharing across boundaries. One Trust showed little progress on either the technical or the social side, with disconnected clusters of low-density relationships. The researchers concluded that the implementation of "lean" is a socio-technical process, and that where collaboration was strong, results from the technical implementation followed (Health Foundation, 2019).

Conclusion

In this chapter we have explored the way in which the mechanistic-scientific orientation has profoundly influenced management and organisational thinking in the 19th and 20th centuries. Scientific management strongly echoes the overarching themes of modernism through its focus on bureaucratic rationality, efficiency and the pursuit of truth. According to Cummings (2002), this is due, at least in part, to the general lack of a critique of the fundamental presuppositions underlying the modernist foundation of organisation and management – the implications of which we will explore in depth in later chapters in this book. This perspective is supported by Stacey and Mowles (2016) who associate it with the prevailing rationalist viewpoint that continues to place a great deal of weight behind the idea of linear causality despite a wealth of evidence to the contrary. This takes us full circle to the teaching of Deming on Theory of Knowledge; that evidence alone does not overcome the beliefs, such as linear causality, that dominate both clinical and non-clinical leadership approaches to change.

Additionally, it could be argued that most efforts to establish quality as the guiding principle in organisations or larger systems have always been constrained by the unconscious consequences of the rationalist model of scientific management. Add to this the ways in which scientific management's simplistic focus on efficiency and productivity, which are often viewed as components of the same thing, has been "cherry-picked" and combined with tools and techniques, particularly those targeted at reducing waste. In many cases, these approaches have been seen to have real benefits on certain types of bounded process problems – especially in the more defined work of secondary care during early years of adoption – although the success is arguably harder to maintain year on year as the "low hanging fruit" has all been harvested. As a result, some of the quality approach's subtler and more difficult philosophical components have become invisible. Many people involved in the quality movement have criticised these notions, arguing that they are fundamentally at odds with the intricate and interconnected nature of the relational work necessary to support people to thrive in their work. It has been argued that many QI projects and programmes have been severely hampered by the lack of well-considered programme theories and rigorous approaches to evaluation (Dixon-Woods

et al., 2013) and thus it has been difficult for quality thinkers to present a sufficiently compelling argument to reset the frame. Perhaps part of this difficulty lies in
the conceptualisation of "the system", which still uses a frame where the individual
and not the relational is seen as the primary unit of interest.

As we progress in this book, we will outline a socio-culturally informed approach
which recognises the critical role that social processes play in supporting quality
and quality improvement, beginning in the next chapter with an exploration of
cultures of quality.

References

Anderson-Wallace, M. 2017. Working with structure. In E. Peck, (ed.), *Organisational
Development in Healthcare* (pp. 167–186). CRC Press.

Anderson-Wallace, M., Blantern, C. and Boydell, T. 2001. Advances in cross-boundary
practice: Inter-logics as method. *Career Development International*, 6(7): 414–420.

Aravind, M. and Chung, K.C. 2010. Evidence-based medicine and hospital reform:
Tracing origins back to Florence Nightingale. *Plastic and Reconstructive Surgery*,
125(1): 403.

Aveling, E.L., Martin, G., Armstrong, N., Banerjee, J. and Dixon-Woods, M. 2012.
Quality improvement through clinical communities: Eight lessons for practice.
Journal of Health Organization and Management, 26(2): 158–174.

Baker, A. 2001. *Crossing the Quality Chasm: A New Health System for the 21st Century.*
British Medical Journal Publishing Group.

Benford, R.D., Hunt, S.A., Holstein, J.A. and Miller, G. 2003. Challenges and choices:
Constructionist perspectives on social problems. *Interactional Dynamics in Public
Problems Marketplaces: Movements and the Counterframing and Reframing of Public
Problems,* pp. 153–160.

Berwick, D. 2008. A transatlantic review of the NHS at 60. *BMJ*, 337: 212. www.bmj.
com/bmj/section-pdf/186530?path=/bmj/337/7663/Analysis.full.pdf

Berwick, D. 2016. Remembering our roots: The intellectual foundations of modern
improvement. IHI Conference, Gothenburg, (13–16 April 2016), Sweden.

Berwick, D., Godfrey, B.A. and Roessner, J. 1991. Curing health care: New strategies
for quality improvement. *The Journal for Healthcare Quality (JHQ)*, 13(5): 65–66.

Blumenthal, D. and Kilo, C.M. 1998. A report card on continuous quality improvement. *The Milbank Quarterly*, 76(4): 625–648.

Blumenthal, D. and Scheck, A.C. 1995. Improving clinical practice: total quality management and the physician, pp. 156–160.

Boaden, R., Harvey, G., Moxham, C. and Proudlove, N. 2008. *Quality Improvement:
Theory and Practice in Healthcare*. NHS Institute for Innovation and Improvement.

Bosshardt, W. and Lopus, J. 2013. Business in the Middle Ages: What was the role of
guilds? *Social Education*, 77(2): 64–67.

Bowns, I.R. and McNulty, T. 1999. *Re-engineering Leicester Royal Infirmary. An Independent Evaluation of Implementation and Impact*. School of Health and Related Research,
University of Sheffield.

Boyne, G.A. and Walker, R.M. 2002. Total quality management and performance: An evaluation of the evidence and lessons for research on public organizations. *Public Performance & Management Review*, 26(2): 111–131.

Britain, G. and Darzi A. 2008. *High Quality Care for All: NHS Next Stage Review Final Report*. Stationery Office.

Burgess, N., Currie, G., Crump, B. and Dawson, A. 2022. *Leading Change Across a Healthcare System: How to Build Improvement Capability and Foster a Culture of Continuous Improvement*. Warwick Business School. https://warwick.ac.uk/fac/soc/wbs/research/vmi-nhs/reports/

Burgess, N., Currie, G., Crump, B., Richmond, J.G. and Johnson, M. (2019) Improving together: Collaboration needs to start with regulators. *BMJ*, 367: 16392.

Cummings, S. 2002. Recreating strategy. *ReCreating Strategy* (pp.1–354). Sage.

Dahlgaard, J.J. and Mi Dahlgaard-Park, S. 2006. Lean production, six sigma quality, TQM and company culture. *The TQM Magazine*, 18(3): 263–281.

Deming, W.E. 2018a. *Out of the Crisis*, reissue. MIT Press.

Deming, W.E. 2018b. *The New Economics* (3rd edn). The MIT Press.

Dixon-Woods, M., Leslie, M., Tarrant, C. and Bion, J. 2013. Explaining Matching Michigan: An ethnographic study of a patient safety program. *Implementation Science*, 8(1): 1–13.

Donabedian, A. 1966. Evaluating the quality of medical care. *The Milbank Memorial Fund Quarterly*, 44(3): 166–206.

Fayol, H. 1916. General principles of management. *Classics of Organization Theory*, 2(15): 57–69.

Gantt, H.L. and Taylor, F. 2007. The pioneers of scientific management. *AACE International Transactions*, PS151–PS153.

Gilbreth, F.B. 1912. *Primer of Scientific Management*. D. Van Nostrand Company.

Ham, C., Kipping, R., McLeod, H. and Meredith, P. 2002. *Capacity, Culture and Leadership: Lessons from Experience of Improving Access to Hospital Services*. Health Services Management Centre. University of Birmingham.

Health Foundation. 2019. *Making Time to Talk*. www.health.org.uk/news-and-comment/blogs/making-time-to-talk-the-challenge-of-spreading-knowledge

Hendricks, K.B. and Singhal, V.R. 2000. The impact of total quality management (TQM) on financial performance: Evidence from quality award winners. *Quality Progress*, 33(4): 35–42.

Hendricks, K.B. and Singhal, V.R. 2001. Firm characteristics, total quality management, and financial performance. *Journal of Operations Management*, 19(3): 269–285.

Horton, R. 2008. The Darzi vision: Quality, engagement, and professionalism. *The Lancet*, 372(9632): 3–4.

Jones, D. and Womack, J. 2003. *Lean Thinking* (1st edn). Simon & Schuster UK Ltd.

Kilo, C.M. 1998. A framework for collaborative improvement: Lessons from the Institute for Healthcare Improvement's Breakthrough Series. *Quality Management in Healthcare*, 6(4): 1–14.

Leape, L.L., Kabcenell, A., Berwick, D.M. and Roessner, J. 1998. *Reducing Adverse Drug Events and Medical Errors*. Institute for Healthcare Improvement.

Lovallo, D. and Kahnerman, D. (2003) *Delusions of Success: How Optimism Undermines Executive's Decisions*. HBR July 2003.

Mayo, E. 1933. The Hawthorne experiment. Western electric company. 2016). Classics of organization theory (pp.134–141). Cengage Learning.

McLeod, H. 2005. A review of the evidence on organisational development in healthcare. Organisational Development in Healthcare: Approaches, innovations, achievements (pp.246–272). Radcliffe.

McLeod, H. and Peck, E. 2005. A review of the evidence on OD in healthcare. In E. Peck (ed.), *Organisational Development in Healthcare: An Introduction.* (pp. 247–261). Radcliffe.

McNulty, T. and Ferlie, E. 2004. Process transformation: Limitations to radical organizational change within public service organizations. *Organization Studies*, 25(8): 1389–1412.

Micklethwaite, J. and Wooldridge, A. 1996. *The Witch Doctors: Making Sense of the Management Gurus.* Heinemann, London.

Mintzberg, H. 1979. *The Structuring of Organizations: A Synthesis of Research.* Prentice-Hall.

Mittman, B.S. 2004. Creating the evidence base for quality improvement collaboratives. *Annals of Internal Medicine*, 140(11): 897–901.

Morgan, G. 1996. *Images of Organization* (New international edn). Sage Publications.

Nelson-Peterson, D.L. and Leppa, C.J. 2007. Creating an environment for caring using lean principles of the Virginia Mason Production System. *JONA: The Journal of Nursing Administration*, 37(6): 287–294.

NHS England Improvement Hub, n.d. *Productive Series.* www.england.nhs.uk/improvement-hub/productives/

Ohno, T. 2019. *Toyota Production System: Beyond Large-Scale Production.* Productivity Press.

Øvretveit, J. and Gustafson, D. 2003. Using research to inform quality programmes. *BMJ*, 326(7392): 759–761.

Øvretveit, J., Bate, P., Cleary, P., Cretin, S., Gustafson, D., McInnes, K., McLeod, H., Molfenter, T., Plsek, P., Robert, G., Shortell, S. and Wilson, T. 2002. Quality collaboratives: Lessons from research. *Quality and Safety in Health Care*, 11: 345–351.

Pettigrew, A., Ferlie, E. and McKee, L. 1992. Shaping Strategic Change: The Case of the NHS in the 1980s. *Public Money & Management*, 12(3): 27–31.

Pugh, D.S., Hinings, C.R. and Hickson, D.J. 1971. *Writers on Organizations* (2nd edn). Penguin Books.

Sarre, S., Robert, G., Maben, J., Griffiths, P. and Chable, R. 2020. Productive Ward ten years on–lessons from a quality improvement programme. *Nursing Times*, 116(3): 27–29.

Shortell, S.M., Bennett, C.L. and Byck, G.R. 1998. Assessing the impact of continuous quality improvement on clinical practice: What it will take to accelerate progress. *The Milbank Quarterly*, 76(4): 593–624.

Stacey, R. and Mowles, C. 2016. *Strategic Management and Organisational Dynamics: The Challenge of Complexity to Ways of Thinking about Organisations.* Pearson.

Strachey, L. 2013. *The Biography of Florence Nightingale.* Simon and Schuster.

Taylor, F.W. 2004. *Scientific Management.* Routledge.

Williams, B. et al. 2019. Evaluation of the impact of an augmented model of The Productive Ward: Releasing Time to Care on staff and patient outcome: A naturalistic stepped wedge trial. *BMJ Quality and Safety*, 30(1): 27–37.

3

Cultures of Quality

┤ Framing ├

In this chapter, we will consider how adopting a cultural lens for considering quality can assist us in effective change. We consider how taking this view of quality can enable us access to a wider vocabulary and repertoire of approaches, methods and techniques for intervention. We will illustrate this through three examples of improvement work that have adopted this approach.

Defining Culture

There has been considerable debate about the term "culture" even amongst scholars in the communities of sociology and anthropology, where the term has its origins. That said, several primary concepts are frequently referred to in the literature, which at the highest level include:

1. The way in which meaning is made in groups (sometimes referred to as the systems of meaning)
2. The way in which societies (from kinship groups to wider communities) organise themselves in relation to these systems of meaning

3. The distinctive techniques that evolve for maintaining, reinforcing, developing and changing things within and between societies

(Adapted from Anderson-Wallace & Blantern, 2005)

Of course, the term "culture" is used in a variety of ways and has wide meaning in our everyday language. We frequently use the terms to describe behaviour, ways of thinking, languages, symbols of status, modes of politeness, prevailing beliefs and unspoken assumptions (Anderson-Wallace & Blantern, 2005). We draw on all those meanings in this chapter.

Whilst this chapter does not allow for an extensive debate of notions of culture, one distinction from the literature is important to make. This relates to whether we treat culture as:

- a **critical variable** in organisational life, which can be manipulated and changed in the same way we might treat structures and technologies

or in contrast,

- the **root metaphor** approach, which rejects the idea that organisations *have a culture* in an objective sense, but are understood as *being cultures*, that is to say that they are the context in which all organisational activity is understood (Schmirch, 1983).

This distinction is important because the chosen orientation has an enormous impact on how people work with issues of culture.

As the Japanese companies of the 1980s and 1990s, many inspired by the work of W. Edwards Deming (referred to in Chapter 2), began to significantly out-perform their North American counterparts in terms of quality, cost and growth, their cultures were seen as a difference that made the difference. Inevitably, this generated a great deal of interest, and programmes focused on culture change based on the critical variable approach were promoted by the large management consultancies and influential business schools. Attempts were made to identify, translate and transplant the cultural, technical (tools) and process strengths of one company to another in the hope that similar performance would follow. Although the approach was presented as scientific, there was little solid research or evidence to support the claims that were made. Nevertheless, the ideas took hold and the notion of "shared values" became the focus of a great deal of work. Strong, powerful and positive cultures became associated with unified, aligned and stable organisations. These "good" cultures were those that were seen to be tight knit and demonstrated a high degree of conformity and commonality (Cummings, 2002). The narrative was compelling, and many organisations committed to large-scale cultural change programmes based on this model. These companies often created a sense of progress, but the results were often unsustainable, focused on process over culture and the correlation between strength of culture and performance seems questionable at best. The critical variable approach is consistent with the scientific paradigm that assumes that the relational social world can be defined in terms of distinct interacting variables within a living subsystem, and that culture can be changed by human influence on the organizational environment (Anderson-Wallace & Blantern, 2005).

Bate (1994) observes the poor record of culture change programmes driven by the critical variable approach, pointing out that:

> such programmatic approaches to culture change rarely speak directly to people's concerns, purposes and aspirations and although a few mission statement and indoctrination sessions might change the senior management's perspective, they are unlikely to lead to sustainable changes in the way that people work, think and relate to each other. (Bate, 1994)

In contrast, the root metaphor approach sees organisations as "societies writ small" (p. 12) and, therefore, cultures (plural) become a metaphor for the total work of the organisation and not just a component of it (Bate, 1994, citing Silverman, 1970). Cultures are the organisation providing a lens through which to interpret the richness of organisational life. Importantly, the root metaphor notion leads to quite different conclusions about improvement practice. If organisations are viewed as cultures, then all improvement work is, de facto, cultural work. As Bate (1994) would have it when using this lens, the task for the improver is "not to think about culture but to think culturally" (Bate, 1994, p. 14). For Bate it is the concept of organisation that is emergent and produced, rather than a monolithic structure that can be viewed as the object of study.

During the late 20th century numerous frameworks and classifications of culture emerged, many driven particularly by the rapidly expanding field of organisational learning and development. One of the most famous of these – and a model that we believe has great utility if treated lightly – was based on the work of Edgar Schein (1990). Schein specifies three layers of culture:

Layer one: *Artefacts* – These are the most visible manifestations of cultures, they include the signs and symbols, rituals and rewards. They also include the architecture, environment and the technologies employed, as well as the meaning that is embodied in uniforms, clothes, manners of address and other codified examples of values and behaviours that are expected. They also include the mythology and stories told about the organisation. Whilst these may be easy to observe (if you are looking) they are often the least noticed, and the task of interpreting the meaning of the artefacts, or whether they are congruent with the espoused values and underlying assumptions of the organisation, can be even harder. Healthcare environments are rich with examples of this layer of culture from the design of facilities – e.g. we provide "waiting rooms" implying that waiting is to be expected – to uniforms, lanyards and badges. It also includes the hierarchies that are implied in job titles and forms of address (formality of Mr or Miss for consultant surgeons even within teams that have worked together for years), and of course the paraphernalia of clinical equipment in consulting environments, even though they are rarely used and many consultations simply involve talking to people.

Layer two: *Espoused values* – These are the values that are used to justify behaviour, decisions and action. They have a clear moral undertone and convey "what ought to be" rather than necessarily "what is". Examples in healthcare range from ethical and professional codes of practice to organisational values and mission statements. We will have all worked in organisations where there feels to be a significant difference between the story told and the story lived when it comes to espoused values, and this dissonance can become problematic. Nevertheless, it can also be an area for rich discussion, and a dynamic and important space to air differences and to evolve new stories and patterns.

Layer three: *Underlying assumptions* – These are the unspoken and often unconscious beliefs and expectations that are collectively shared. They are seen as representing the truth about the world; the things that are taken for granted and the areas of organisational life where to behave in any other way would be unthinkable. Because of this these assumptions are not debated or confronted, and hence are difficult to change. According to Schein, only values that are susceptible to validation and continue to work reliably in solving the group's problems will become transformed into underlying assumptions. In healthcare, we might consider the Hippocratic Oath or "First do no harm" as an example of such an underlying assumption, or issues of confidentiality or that healthcare professionals should not prescribe medicines for themselves or for members of their own families.

There are many complexities associated with the way this model is presented, not least being the neat and rational way in which such a complex issue is described. However, the model provides at least some structure to explain and then explore the notion of cultures, especially to those who think of it as too "woolly" or inaccessible to be an area worth consideration. We use this principle of exploring underlying and often unsaid assumptions as one of the methods for questioning the work to improve quality in later chapters in this book.

Cultures of Care

In the wake of every quality scandal in healthcare – ranging from Ely Hospital in the 1950s to more recent events at Mid Staffordshire, East Kent, Shrewsbury and Telford Hospitals (and sadly there will inevitably be more in the future) we hear the rallying call for a "change in culture" – but we rarely spend any time considering exactly what is meant by this. The default position therefore tends to be the critical variable approach to culture, which promotes the idea that we can "fix" cultural problems in the way that we might replace a specific component on a faulty household appliance. This reflects both the wider rationalist thinking that is still prevalent in healthcare policy, and the expediency in our politics. If we adopt the root metaphor approach however, the picture is more complex and messier, and the responsibility for change is shared more widely. This is because we start to see the organisations – or to be more precise the ways of organising – as an expression of the cultures that are creating the problems. This is not about the often tempting and neat notion of individuals or "rotten apples", it is about the broader systemic context and how relations are being enacted at multiple levels.

Following the Mid Staffs scandal, Anderson-Wallace and Shale (2013) identified three traps, as a warning to those who were preparing to address the "cultural problems" identified within the report of the Public Inquiry (Francis, 2013).

- The first trap draws attention to the risk of adopting a view that things were better in the past and that NHS culture is "a descent from compassion to depravity". Whilst the dominant media stories might strongly suggest this, any historical examination of healthcare practice shows us something quite different – that in the NHS at least, the population's health, safety and outcomes are better now than in the past. Of course, the expectations we place on healthcare and the standards of care that have consequently emerged are radically different from the past, and a great deal of evolution – often imperceptible over time – has occurred. The mourning of a lost utopia is therefore fallacious.
- The second trap is the belief that culture alone determines what people do. There are plenty of studies in social psychology that show us this, but the seminal study most often cited to illustrate this is that of the Good Samaritan (Darley & Batson, 1973). Conducted at Princeton Theological College, students were invited to participate in a study of religious vocation – based on the story of the Good Samaritan. Once they had completed a standard personality questionnaire, the students were invited to make a presentation on the theme, which was to take place in a different building on campus. A third of the group were told they were early; a third were told that they were on time; and a third that they were late. Each group set off to the other campus building and en route encountered a person slumped on the ground. It was unclear if the person was hurt or drunk, but they were in obvious distress. The majority of those who were in a hurry because they thought they were late carried on and ignored the need for help, whereas the vast majority of those running early stopped to give assistance. Darley and Batson claimed that what was learnt from this experiment was that neither "culture" nor "character" were reliable predictors of who will offer help when needed. There was nothing inherently "wrong" with the culture of the seminary, and there were no specific character defects in the students from the group who thought they were late – indeed they were assigned entirely randomly. The difference between them and their apparently more altruistic peers was the way that the task they had been given was framed, and the interaction between this and the context.

If we translate this learning to a healthcare environment it draws our attention to how groups of practitioners define their work and how they signal to each other what is important as members of the same moral community. If the task is to get through a list of tasks, and people who need help are impediments to that, then do not expect compassionate results. If the task, however, is to demonstrate effective, personalised and safe care, and people who need help are opportunities to do exactly that, then it might be reasonable to think that things will turn out better.

- The third trap is that of thinking that culture is monolithic. As discussed in our consideration of the critical variable approach to culture, if we treat "it" as a single coherent object, a component part that we can manipulate, upgrade or re-engineer as if it were a faulty part in a machine, then our responses will be mechanical rather than human.

Instead, it is more pragmatically useful to think of healthcare as having many cultures, which arise dynamically from the multiplicity of exceptions, assumptions and beliefs that are expressed in the day-to-day patterns of interaction between all those involved. Now this is not to say that each actor shapes the interactions equally as we know that power dynamics have a significant role to play. Indeed, in healthcare, regulatory frameworks and professional standards, political ideologies and societal trends and many other emergent factors play a huge part in shaping the cultural norms, and these may differ from place to place, and even from day to day.

Building Clinical Communities

Mary Dixon-Woods and colleagues (2013), citing Greenhalgh et al. (2004), discuss how those in charge of quality improvement programmes have gradually but steadily started to recognise the importance of comprehending the cultural dimensions of change. Citing Grol and Grimshaw (2003) they specifically highlight the need to give attention to particularly the social processes of QI programmes to counter the "unhelpful and pervasive tendency to conceptualise the diffusion-uptake process as a technical-rational, linear process that is simply about putting into practice predefined strategies for changing (individual) clinicians' behaviours" (Grol & Grimshaw, 2003, p. 1227). Clinical communities that function well, according to this argument, are characterised by "careful balancing of bottom-up, localising, participatory and informal social processes and strong leadership, coordination and impetus from within – and sometimes from beyond or even 'above'" (Aveling et al., 2012, p.162). This advice comes with a warning that the benefits of clinical communities in the QI context can be easily destabilised, and that those attempting to structure the work must proceed with extreme caution and consideration to make sure their input does not undermine the very traits that positively set clinical communities apart. Importantly, they caution against the search for overarching "laws" of success by pointing out the variety of approaches and contexts in which improvement work has been attempted. They emphasise taking time to build a clear "theory of change", investing in building social capital across boundaries, and attention to a range of what we might describe as relational leadership sensibilities (Malby & Anderson-Wallace, 2016; Oliver, 2018).

Cultural Interventions

Although there are many examples we could choose to illustrate how some of these ideas have been put into practice, we have chosen to highlight three. The reason for this is because of the emphasis these initiatives put on what we might call the cultural patterns and practices, and where the focus was on building cultures of quality. All of them seemed to recognise that the most significant element of the change achieved in their contexts was fundamental shifts in belief systems, in basic shared assumptions and ideologies, and not just the technical or expert driven change. The work also entered the ethical and moral domain, where the changes they were making were focused on shifting the normative expectations of a clinical community, changing the norms, assumptions and expectations, and redefining standards of behaviour and building the relationship between meaning and action over time.

The first of these is the Keystone Project in Michigan, led by Dr Peter Pronovost, an Intensive Care Unit (ICU) doctor. The aim of the work was to completely eradicate central venous catheter (CVC) bloodstream infections during the insertion and use of central lines. This is a frequent practice in critical and intensive care environments and involves the insertion of a device used to draw blood and give treatments, including intravenous fluids, drugs or blood transfusions. A thin, flexible tube is inserted into a vein, usually below the collarbone. It is guided into a large vein above the right side of the heart. A CVC may stay in place for weeks or months and helps avoid the need for repeated use of needles. The risk of infection is high and therefore great care must be taken to prevent this. Infections have profound consequences and could be fatal. Whilst clearly undesirable, a level of infection was accepted as a normal complication of the procedure. Pronovost however was unwilling to accept this and like Semmelweiss in the 19th century (discussed in Chapter 2) demonstrated through careful observation and collection of data that a specific set of actions performed reliably as a combination – referred to as "a bundle" – could dramatically reduce and ultimately eradicate these infections. What Pronovost and his colleagues showed was that the belief that a level of infection was inevitable was unfounded, and he set out to eradicate CVC infections not only in his unit, but also across the whole state of Michigan. The project was designed using a large-scale collaborative approach (Mills & Weeks, 2004; Øvretveit et al., 2002). It was not achieved through mandates or through regulation, but by a collegiate peer-based approach, which shifted the clinical and cultural practices of the people working in those ICUs.

The intervention was widely reported in the popular media as being the triumph of a simple checklist (Bosk et al., 2009) but the reality of the intervention was vastly different. As Dixon-Woods et al. (2011) attest it was in fact a complex social intervention involving a detailed theory of change. In their excellent ex-post theoretical account of the programme, six reasons to explain why the programme succeeded were identified.

- Firstly, the programme team created "isomorphic" pressures, both within and between the state's ICUs. Isopmorphism is a sociological concept, which when applied to organisations provides an explanation of the "forces" that lead to them resembling one another. Three main forces – the normative, coercive and memetic – are seen to influence behaviour and practice. Simply put, organisations conform because they believe it to be the "right" thing to do (normative); they do so because they are coerced by rules and regulations (coercive), or they aim to copy others to become more like them (mimetic) (DiMaggio & Powell, 1983). Although it sounds relatively simple, the interplay between these forces is complex, and the balance is particularly important. Some coercive pressures were noted in the Michigan programme, but they were seen to be primarily normative and mimetic.
- Secondly, a rich and complex networked community was built, developing peer and coaching relationships, with educational interventions to support technical changes. This "sense of community" became strong, and the design of workshops included highly active and purposeful development of social relations among members. There was significant focus on the development of horizontal relationships across boundaries, especially to support informal problem solving and sharing of "know-how". But the approach to networking was not entirely "bottom-up" and involved a good degree of strong internal direction and top-down leadership, much of which was focused on creating the conditions to enable participation. Cornish (2006) notes this combination of both horizontal and vertical integration is noted as being important for quality improvement communities, in order to coordinate activity and manage potentially competing interests.
- Thirdly, the bloodstream infections were reframed as a social problem that could be solved, and not purely a technical matter. By disrupting the norms and behaviour of the community through a combination of persuasion and "meaning work" (Benford & Snow, 2000; Benford et al., 2003) infection was also positioned as a problem that could and must be solved. The combination of the possibility for change and the moral imperative was powerfully amplified using compelling patient stories to vividly illustrate the human cost of the avoidable harm. This qualitative data was skilfully combined with the quantitative, which also showed levels of unwarranted variation in infections across

units. This in turn began to create a story that risked discrediting ICUs as "safe places" and thereby constructing an uncomfortable professional identity for ICU staff. This was considered to be a pivotal process, which could have created defensiveness and additional anxiety, but seemed to have a motivating effect.

- Fourthly, the invention involved defined goals to make change at the "sharp end" of clinical and cultural practice. Logistical, operational, financial and administrative support for the interventions was also made available. This gave the intervention significant meaning, both through the practical organisational support, but also strong relevance in daily practice. A five point locally adapted checklist was developed and a peer-based system of observation and feedback was initiated. Compliance with the checklist was monitored carefully and supportively with the aim of helping to build a sense of collective responsibility for outcomes. The checklist was framed as a supporting mechanism to assist people in doing "the right thing" both clinically and morally. Using the PDSA cycle was suggested, but not enforced, which Dixon-Woods et al. suggests meant that the presence of a strong programme theory may have been more influential than the tools and techniques normally associated with QI.
- Fifthly, the programme harnessed data on infection as a disciplinary force. The systematic collection of data was centralised, but not made public. Dixon-Woods et al. (2011) emphasise the importance and fatefulness of the process of measurement, citing Latour (1987) who notes that as we measure phenomena and events, and translate them into data to enable evaluation, comparison and intervention, the system of measurement acts on the system being measured and creates its own effects as a non-human actor in the network of relationships. The issue of data collection is therefore a complex one and far from neutral.
- Finally, although consensus, community building and consent were huge components of the programme's success, skilful use of what were described as the "hard edges" was also noted. They relied on a level of force from the new social norms, and the possible social sanction of "loss of face". The latent supervisory effect of the checklist was thought to enhance procedural accountability by "leaving a trace" and potentially increasing staff commitment to their performance to avoid censure later. They also employed "activist tactics" to ensure co-operation. For example, the failure to submit data to the programme risked a call to the CEO with a request for the same, which if not forthcoming then led to an invitation to leave. No hospitals left the programme.

It is noted that the detailed analysis of the theory undertaken in the Michigan work is rare within most QI work in healthcare. It could be argued that the lack of understanding of QI work as complex socio-cultural interventions is part of the reason that transferability is often poor, and that although learning can take place, outcomes can be disappointing even when local adaptations are made. In conclusion, Dixon-Woods et al. identify several valuable lessons for QI more generally. First, they contend that while isomorphic effects can explain why people joined the programme, this can backfire if only a few organisations become "beacons" or "showcases"; instead, they advise involving a large number of organisations and letting mimetic or normative forces take control.

Second, they stress the value of creating a sense of community and investing in peer relationships, but they also emphasise the need for a strong vertical core to coordinate and support, particularly during inevitable periods of significant challenge. Having a thorough understanding of the social forces that can make or break a programme seems essential, but is frequently lacking in poorly thought out and underfunded QI initiatives. The restructuring of working relationships is their ultimate point for attention, noting vulnerability because new rituals and patterns of behaviour frequently – and necessarily – put existing authority structures and power dynamics to the test. Being aware of these tensions and conflicts that new power relations might create requires forethought and supportive processes to enable them to be worked through.

Our second example, which also involves the introduction of a checklist, but this time on a global level, shares several significant similarities with the Michigan programme. The work was led by Atul Gawande, a professor at Harvard Medical School and a surgeon at Boston's Brigham and Women's Hospital. The checklist was created and promoted by the World Health Organization and like Pronovost's checklist for BSI CVC infections, this seemingly straightforward technology brought to light several important socio-cultural practices within the surgical environment, especially those connected to traditional patterns of authority and hierarchical practices.

Gawande's work brought attention to the crucial – and frequently extremely uncomfortable – cultural aspects of clinical practice in surgery, particularly in relation to fundamental dynamics of inclusion and exclusion, respect for others, and basic communication.

These areas were felt to prevent communication, normalise deviation and subsequently increase surgical error and complication. Despite being used globally, the WHO surgical checklist has not consistently reduced the error incidents it was intended to address. These so-called "Never Events" in surgery have, in fact, proven to be incredibly stubborn in some places, and this is thought to be related to a variety of complex socio-cultural dimensions that are local, situated and contextual (Aveling et al., 2013). According to the research, the effects of the checklist are likely to be maximised regardless of the environments, when an extensive organisational and cultural programme to improve safety is also being implemented. They point out that it certainly cannot be assumed that the checklist will improve clinical procedures and communication on its own.

Our final example is at the healthcare system level and focuses on the NUKA system of care developed by the Southcentral Foundation, a not-for-profit healthcare provider based in Anchorage, Alaska. The NUKA system is considered to provide a model of care provision that breaches many of the conventional taken-for-granted approaches in healthcare provision, and thus is a cultural intervention at scale

(Anderson-Wallace, 2017; Gottlieb, 2013). In 2014, Professor Don Berwick commented that NUKA was the leading example of healthcare redesign in the world, stating that he believed that in future we will look back on the NUKA system and see them as pathfinders who led healthcare globally to a "new and proper destination". The NUKA system is regarded to be one of the highest quality and the lowest cost healthcare systems in the world (Baker, 2011) and is three-time winner of the Malcolm Baldridge Award for Quality, an award frequently won by much larger and more prestigious healthcare, industrial and commercial organisations in the US.

The genesis of the NUKA system is an important context. During the 1980s the Alaskan native community had become very dissatisfied by educational and healthcare systems that were being provided by the Federal Government as part of the settlement with native communities. The quality of services were poor, delays were long, access to care – particularly in primary care – was very problematic and population health outcomes were amongst the worst in the whole of the USA. The costs of this inferior quality of care were rising significantly. The Alaska Native community therefore negotiated to take over the running of services from the Indian Health Services (a large bureaucratic entity set up by the Federal Government). The budget was set; it could not cost more than the current arrangements, and ideally should cost less.

The Alaska Native Community got to work purposefully creating services in a completely new mould after realising that nothing short of radical reform would make this possible.

This process started with a thorough listening exercise to fully comprehend the needs and priorities of the local population. The NUKA system that emerged is characterised by a clear focus on kinship and family wellness, as well as shared accountability and responsibility for health and wellbeing between "customer-owners" and those who provide care.

Most of the population's health services are provided by Southcentral Foundation on a prepaid/free at the point of delivery basis.

The NUKA system is based on the fundamental tenet that the majority of healthcare delivery occurs in the "complex adaptive" space; that is, that care is neither so unpredictable or novel as to require significant intuitive innovation nor is it sufficiently predictable as to warrant a wholly standardised or protocolised approach. Although NUKA acknowledges the need for a variety of interventions, they have concluded after giving the health needs of their population careful consideration that most resources should go towards low acuity, chronic, and frequently complex care. This is based on the pragmatic assumption that the level of acuity has a significant impact on the control of outcomes; where acuity is high, professionals have more influence, but where acuity is lower, patient and families have most impact (Eby, 2018).

NUKA is built on a small set of simple and yet intensely human beliefs. At its core, the system aims to reconnect people into the web of life as the primary focus of all healthcare interventions. The approach is fundamentally relational. But NUKA is not just a warm, humanist idea. It has produced tangible results in the areas where the NHS really struggles. In the first 10 years of operation, SCF experienced a 40% reduction in A&E services, a 50% drop in referrals to specialists and a decrease in primary care visits by 20%. At the same time overall health outcomes for the population improved and staff satisfaction is exceptional. It has continued to see significant improvements in quality of care within the constraints of limited finance. By producing significant improvements in quality of services, costs have reduced and demand for services has fallen. Perhaps most significantly, the cost of care – unlike all other healthcare systems in developed countries – is not increasing. Interestingly, SCF did not set out with those objectives in mind. They did not chase the numbers, nor did they set targets. They designed a relational system that was congruent with and supportive of their values. They focused on providing care that was responsive to the emergent needs and wishes of their communities. They placed their beliefs and values in the foreground and had the courage of their convictions to see it through. Of course, this has all taken time and NUKA has been serving the native Alaskan community for more than 30 years, but its strongly relational focus, which is culturally appropriate and resonant with the values and beliefs of the native population, appears to have paid dividends. Importantly, NUKA chose to work on the issues that most deeply affected their communities, which involved a substantial investment in trauma-informed approaches, including innovative programmes to work with the effects of domestic abuse and sexual violence, which plagued their communities. They also focused on culturally sensitive programmes for young men afflicted by depression, alcohol and drug misuse and high rates of death by suicide, aimed at recovering a sense of purpose and identity to combat generations of cultural alienation and epistemic exclusion.

Many features of the NUKA system – philosophically, aesthetically and in clinical practice – can also be seen in the pioneering design of some of the 1920s pre-NHS health centres in the UK. Rather than focusing on individual pathology, these services were interested in understanding the patterns of ill health and disease within their communities. Today, we still see some examples of such practice in Healthy Living Centres such as Bromley-by-Bow in London; Bunnyhill in Sunderland; and the Wester Hailes Project in Edinburgh with other local examples beginning to slowly emerge in other areas of the UK. At the heart of all these services lies a belief that the quality of relationships (between users and professionals as well as within families and social support networks) is fundamental to better health outcomes, alongside a keen sense of purpose, meaning and self-determination.

Conclusion

In this chapter we have both defined and discussed notions of culture, and how these can be applied in organisational work to improve quality. What we hope is clear from the examples offered is the critical role that understanding cultures plays in initiating and sustaining improvement work; and how a depth of appreciation and skill is needed to do this work effectively. A strong theme that emerges from the examples offered is also the importance of developing a sound theory of change or programme theory, taking suitable time to think very carefully with others about what and how you think the change happens and building an infrastructure to support this. As we hope this chapter has demonstrated, the disappointing outcomes of many – perhaps even most – quality improvement projects and programmes arise from a lack of attention to these crucial dimensions. Having the technical solution is simply not enough.

References

Anderson-Wallace, M. 2017. Working with structure. In E. Peck (ed.), *Organisational Development in Healthcare: Approaches, Innovations, Achievements* (pp. 167–186). CRC Press.

Anderson-Wallace, M. and Blantern, C. 2005. Working with culture. In E. Peck (ed.), *Organisational Development in Healthcare: Approaches, Innovations, Achievements* (pp. 187–204). CRC Press.

Anderson-Wallace, M. and Shale, S. 2013. Should there be changes to NHS culture? *The Guardian*. www.theguardian.com/healthcare-network/2013/mar/27/changes-nhs-culture-wake-francis

Aveling, E., McCulloch, P. and Dixon-Woods, M. 2013. A qualitative study comparing experiences of the surgical safety checklist in hospitals in high-income and low-income countries. *BMJ Open*, 3: e003039. doi: 10.1136/bmjopen-2013-003039

Aveling, E.L., Martin, G., Armstrong, N., Banerjee, J. and Dixon-Woods, M. 2012. Quality improvement through clinical communities. Eight lessons for practice. *Journal of Health Organisation and Management*, 26(2): 158–174.

Baker, G.R. 2011. *A Comparative Study of Three Transformative Healthcare Systems*. desLibris.

Bate, S.P. 1994. *Strategies for Cultural Change*. Butterworth-Heinneman.

Benford, R.D. and Snow, D.A. 2000. Framing processes and social movements: An overview and assessment. *Annual Review of Sociology*, 26(1): 611–639.

Benford, R.D. and Hunt, S.A. 2003. Interactional dynamics in public problems marketplaces: Movements and the counterframing and reframing of public problems. In J.A. Holstein and G. Miller (ed.), *Challenges and Choices: Constructionist Perspectives on Social Problems* (pp. 153–86). New York: Aldine de Gruyter.

Bosk, C.L., Dixon-Woods, M., Goeschel, C.A. and Pronovost, P.J. 2009. Reality check for checklists. *The Lancet*, 374(9688): 444–445.

Cornish, F. 2006. Empowerment to participate: A case study of participation by Indian sex workers in HIV prevention. *Journal of Community and Applied Social Psychology*, 16(4): 301–315.

Cummings, S. 2002. Recreating strategy. *ReCreating Strategy*, pp. 1–354. Sage.

Darley, J.M. and Batson, C.D. 1973. "From Jerusalem to Jericho": A study of situational and dispositional variables in helping behavior. *Journal of Personality and Social Psychology*, 27(1): 100.

DiMaggio, P.J., and Powell, W.W. 1983. The iron cage revisited: Institutional iso-morphism and collective rationality in organizational fields. *American Sociological Review*, 48(2): 147–160.

Dixon-Woods, M., Bosk, C.L., Aveling, E.L., Goeschel, C.A. and Pronovost, P.J. 2011. Explaining Michigan: Developing an ex-post theory of a quality improvement program. *The Milbank Quarterly*, 89(2): 167–205.

Dixon-Woods, M., Leslie, M., Tarrant, C. and Bion, J. 2013. Explaining Matching Michigan: An ethnographic study of a patient safety program. *Implementation Science*, 8(1): 1–13.

Eby, D.K. 2018. Customer-ownership in equity-oriented health care. *The Milbank Quarterly*, 96(4): 672.

Francis, R. 2013. *Report of the Mid Staffordshire NHS Foundation Trust Public Inquiry: Executive Summary* (Vol. 947). The Stationery Office.

Gottlieb, K. 2013. The NUKA System of Care: Improving health through ownership and relationships. *International Journal of Circumpolar Health*, 72(1): 21118.

Greenhalgh, T., Robert, G., Macfarlane, F., Bate, P. and Kyriakidou, O. 2004. Diffusion of innovations in service organizations: Systematic review and recommendations. *The Milbank Quarterly*, 82(4): 581–629.

Grol, R. and Grimshaw, J. 2003. From best evidence to best practice: Effective imple-mentation of change in patients' care. *The Lancet*, 362(9391): 1225–1230.

Horton, R. 2008. The Darzi vision: quality, engagement, and professionalism. *The Lancet*, 372(9632): 3–4.

Latour, B. 1987. *Science in Action*. Open University Press.

Malby, B. and Anderson-Wallace, M. 2016. Leading healthcare networks. In *Networks in Healthcare* (pp. 133–156). Emerald Group Publishing Limited.

Mills, P.D. and Weeks, W.B. 2004. Characteristics of successful quality improvement teams: Lessons from five collaborative projects in the VHA. *Joint Commission Jour-nal on Quality and Patient Safety*, 30(3): 152–162.

Oliver, C. 2018. *Reflexive Inquiry: A Framework for Consultancy Practice*. Routledge.

Øvretveit, J., Bate, P., Cleary, P., Cretin, S., Gustafson, D., McInnes, K., McLeod, H., Molfenter, T., Plsek, P., Robert, G., Shortell, S. and Wilson, T. 2002. Quality col-laboratives: Lessons from research. *Quality and Safety in Health Care*, 11: 345–351.

Schein, E.H. 1990. *Organizational Culture* (Vol. 45, No. 2, p. 109). American Psycho-logical Association.

Schmirch, L. 1983. Concepts of culture and organizational analysis. *Administrative Science Quarterly*, 28(3): 339–358.

4

Understanding Variation – Tensions and Dilemmas

Framing

In this chapter we will set out the core principles and considerations on the prominent topic of variation in healthcare and how it can be used to understand quality and question the work. We will peel away the layers of this subject, which at first glance seem simple, but on further exploration have profound implications, many of which are only just beginning to be understood in healthcare. We set out why the concept of variation is so important, the common considerations, analytic methods that help determine when to question the work and the tensions we need to be aware of when we seek to either manage, or in some cases promote variability. We will conclude by discussing setting dependent considerations, and tensions that need to be managed, to achieve quality gains through reducing inappropriate, unwarranted variation.

As first introduced in Chapter 1, we will be using a holistic interpretation when referring to quality in this and subsequent chapters. In quality we mean not only safety and experience, but also mean effectiveness, equity and efficiency – as proposed by the IoM (Institute of Medicine, 2001).

This chapter also marks a slight change in tone from the previous three. From the socio-cultural to the technical. As we have concluded in previous chapters, these should not be viewed as separate, but rather they should co-exist as enablers towards a common goal. That of effective improvement of quality. Despite it being a more technical commentary, it is not written with the assumption of technical or statistical knowledge – it is written with the only prerequisite being that of curiosity and desire to improve services. We aim to make accessible and contextualise what is often off-putting or theoretical in technical texts, and to highlight and draw attention to important issues of application that are frequently overlooked issues in busy healthcare settings.

Variation

Consider a simple exercise that we often run with groups of clinicians. Take a child's toy – a catapult, and ask a group of six people to launch a ball five times each from a defined, set, angle from that catapult. They are using the same equipment, the same angle and the same ball and so you might expect such a group to all be achieving the same distance on each shot. But the capability of the process to deliver the same distance always varies. This is variation in action.

In five minutes, you could list 40 or 50 sources of variation, ranging from how far people pulled the catapult back (was it exactly the defined angle?), changes in how people held the catapult, differences in measurement, differences in interpretation of the task and even, sometimes, a little gaming (cheating) of the exercise. These are all sources of variation. Now consider a process in health or social care. There are hundreds if not thousands of sources of variation. They all have an impact to some degree and all are contributing to *the difference between what is intended and what actually happens* (American Society for Quality, 2020).

As Professor Don Berwick, former CEO of the Institute of Healthcare Improvement and leading quality thinker concludes, variation is also a thief (Berwick, 1991) which robs processes of the qualities they intended to have.

Eugine Litvak and Michael Long describe the proposition of healthcare without variation:

Suppose all patients are homogeneous in disease process. That they all have the same disease, same degree of illness and same response to therapy. Suppose they all appear at a uniform rate. Furthermore, suppose all medical practitioners and provider services have the same ability to deliver quality care. In this scenario it would be possible to deliver the best of care 100% of the time. (Litvak & Long, 2000)

While this panacea to its fullest extent is fiction, you can see that in this world it would be extremely efficient, safety could be maximised and care could be delivered in a well-planned manner that does not burden staff.

What Gets in the Way? - Variation

Variation is also the world of management and leadership. Management is essentially a cycle of hypothesis (Scholtes, 1998). If we do *this* (X – although, given complexity, it is almost never just one thing that needs to change) then we will get *that* (Y) – something desirable like an improvement in quality and productivity. These hypotheses can be in the form of plans, snatched conversations in a corridor or in a formal document like a business case of a report from a management consultancy firm. Our ability as a manager or leader is dependent on the strength of our hypothesis – regardless of whether it is written down in a glossy report or even prepared by a management consultancy – but we often lose sight of this. The strength of our hypothesis is reliant on the understanding of the variables at play, and the variation within those variables. Most fundamentally, a hypothesis is useless unless proven by data (Scholtes, 1998, p. 33).

Understanding Variation

The simple run chart, sometimes called a line chart, is a powerful tool to enable the more informed interpretation of variability. It is the graphical representation of variability data that provides us with the knowledge and thus better improvement decisions that data on its own does not. Most importantly it helps us to determine which bits of the work we should be asking questions of. Much of the interesting information available in your data is tied up in the time-order sequence of values (Poling & Wheeler, 1998) as displayed in a run chart. The simple run chart itself, by substituting the average line for a median line,[1] can be combined with a set of interpretation rules that aid our interpretation and building of knowledge of things like demand profiles and process reliability – especially if we move to collecting and displaying data in this way on an ongoing basis.

These interpretation rules provide us with signals that tell us that something to take notice of is happening with our data; or when to begin to question the work and context. Crucially, the absence of a signal is just as important as the presence of one, as it tells us nothing significant has happened and that the process is stable. So don't rush and change things as it will likely make things worse. This is one of Deming's core teachings in his work *The New Economics* (Deming, 2018).

For a run chart these signals are:

- Six or more points above or below the established median
- Five or more points going in one direction (up or down)

- Non-random patterns. Data should vary with regularity, although not in a pattern, above and below the median line. If not, it is a signal that something of significance has happened
- Astronomical points. Very high or low numbers when considered against the general distribution along the run chart

(Adapted from Murray, et al., 2011)

The useful thing about these run chart interpretation rules is that they are visual prompts. You don't need a degree in maths to either produce a run chart or use the rules to identify signals. They democratise the interpretation of data.

The fact that these signals tell us something significant has happened is important. The rules are helping us identify and distinguish the variation in our data and react appropriately. There are two types of variation at play here. Some of which is predictable and some of which is unpredictable.

Common Cause, Normal, Routine, Chance Cause

Common cause variation is noise. It is *normal* for the process in its current state. These are the expected (to the enlightened, variation aware leader) variations in the process and its outcome. These variations stay the same day to day over a long period of time (Deming, 2018). Multiple sources of variation contribute to variations in process capability. To improve a process that is showing common cause variation, the whole process and its variables need to be taken into account in the improvement strategy.

Example of common cause variation:

Take a ward-based nursing team at lunch times.[2] The team will probably have a figure in their head for how long it takes to give out lunches to all 28 patients on their ward. In this case they have a figure of 30 minutes in their head that allows them to plan their tasks before and after. Sometimes it takes a little longer and sometimes it takes less time. The team probably would not even raise an eyebrow if the meals took 40 minutes to dish out, as this happens so often. Or conversely, they might not notice if it took 20 minutes. This is down to the huge number of sources of variation at play in this scenario. A non-exhaustive list of variations could be:

- The case mix of patients (their dependency)
- The mix of nursing staff (who was working)
- What tasks were outstanding from the morning
- Any visitors on the ward

- The mix of meal types
- Availability of mealtime equipment
- Arrival of the meals
- The morale of the nursing team

The nursing team know that all of these variations are at play and they expect them – but they are so common and subtle that they would not be able to really put their finger on a single source of a particular small increase or decrease in time taken (and might not even notice them) – as they are generally all influencing at some point. The outcome of the process is not attributable to a specific event but is the result of the culmination of multiple contributing factors. The outcome of the process varies every day but is predictable between certain limits (in our case 20 and 40 minutes).

Special Cause, Exceptional, Assignable, Uncontrolled

Special cause variation is where one or more instances of variation are assignable to specific causes. These causes could be particular events, like a lack of a specific consumable on one day or specific shifts in the data – where "runs" of data signal a special cause – as signalled by the run chart signal rules explored previously. For example, a new member of staff who is less familiar with the job starts work. The word *assignable* is important as it suggests you can pinpoint the occurrence and then problem solve the reason (assigning it).

Example of special cause variation:

Returning to our example of mealtimes on a ward. An instance of special cause variation would be if one day the mealtime took 60 minutes. The staff would definitely notice this. During the problem solving that was triggered, it emerged that there was a kitchen ordering problem which affected the meal preparation and a number of incorrect meals arrived. This variation in the overall process time could be assigned to a specific source of special cause variation.

The distinction between the two is vital for managers and leaders. Deming, quoting Shewhart, describes two fundamental mistakes managers make when trying to improve processes:

Mistake one: Reacting to and seeking to improve a process outcome as if it came from special cause (judging it was assignable to a specific event) when in fact it was "just" common cause variation - it was to be expected from the process in its current state.

Mistake two: Reacting to and seeking to improve a process outcome as if it was common cause variation, normal for the process in its current state, when it was not - it was assignable to a specific event.

(Adapted from Deming, 2018, p. 120)

The implication of this is profound. By making mistake one, the common consequence would be to pinpoint a source of the perceived variation and take action – for example taking action against a supplier, individual, team etc. At best this would be ineffective due to the fact it is in fact common cause variation – variation that is normal and predictable for the process in its current state. The only way to improve the process is by viewing the process as a whole with its interlinked web of sources of variation. At worst it introduces another source of special cause variation. The typical resulting action plan, based on the flawed perception of a special cause event, will introduce completely avoidable additional variation – making the process less predictable, not more.

Moving onto mistake two, by mistakenly assuming all the variation is normal, the implication is an entire process may be significantly changed, causing significant upheaval for not only the process but also any up or downstream processes. This huge introduction of variation (unpredictability) could have been avoided as the cause was special – it was assignable to a specific event or issue and thus could have been problem solved in a traditional manner such as root cause analysis.

Statistical Process Control Charts

To provide greater structure for the visual interpretation of the data, the search for signals to differentiate special and common cause variation, a common next step from a run chart is the statistical process control (SPC) chart. This is a form of graphical display of data developed by the great contemporary of Edwards Deming, Walter A. Shewhart, and sometimes referred to as a Shewhart chart. Before we explore the structure of an SPC chart, it is worth re-iterating the value of the run chart. Many managers start from a position of statistical abstinence (Scholtes, 1998). This is the case for many organisations, managers and clinicians alike. Operational decisions are made with no data, little data, poorly presented misleading data or a combination of the three. With this in mind, a huge amount can be gained from progressing to the use of the easy to produce and understand run chart. As will be discussed, an SPC chart is undeniably very useful, and in some applications critical, but they are also more involved to produce – often taking up very scant analytical capacity (if any exists in the first place). You can make enormous first steps in supercharging your use of data to understand and question your work using the run chart – don't delay this step by waiting until you have SPC chart capability across the board.

SPC charts are also sometimes called process capability or process behaviour charts (Poling & Wheeler, 1998, p. 87). This relates to one of the main aims of SPC charts – that of understanding if a process is in statistical control. In other words, whether a process has definable capability (Deming, 2018, p. 67). Having a definable capability gives confidence that it will achieve a certain level of quality, or throughput, or both; vital for planning, vital for costing and most importantly vital for patients. It gives us predictability. It also goes some way to reducing the downstream variation felt by other process steps – it reduces their demand variation.

SPC charts take the same initial format as our run chart. With the time interval on the X axis and, in the case of this demand discussion, the number of referred procedures received per week on the Y axis. With an SPC chart the mean is used instead of the median, and two graphical interpretation guides are calculated. These are called the upper and lower control limits. In this text we are not going to explain how these limits are derived as that is explained in a number of excellent texts.[3] Here we will concentrate on the interpretation of SPC charts and what insights they can bring.

An SPC chart makes the application of the signal rules already discussed easier through the introduction of visual interpretation guides – called control limits. These control limits are set to distinguish the special from common cause variation. They are typically set limits, derived from 3 sigma – that where 99.7% of all data points would be expected to fall within them – the common or normal variation. Anything outside of them is extremely unusual and is a signal for investigation. This provides a powerful clarification to the "astronomical points" signal explored earlier. The identification of what makes an astronomical point can now be exact. It will be outside of the control limits.

The list below details typical further SPC chart special cause variation signal rules:

- Any single point outside the control limits
- A run of seven points all above or below the average
- A run of seven points all consecutively ascending or descending
- The number of points within the middle third of the region between the control limits differs markedly from two thirds of the total number of points (essentially a sustained spread or narrowing of the points)

(ACT Academy, 2020)

A question that is often asked is why do some texts or institutions use the rule of fives as a signal, for example a run of five above the average,[4] and why use the rule of sevens or even eight points to signal possible special cause variation / significant process change? The answer lies in what each says about the probability of something unlikely (special – assignable) happening that each suggests. In other words, the likelihood that the run could only have taken place if something significant had happened in the process (good or bad). Take a coin flip as a simplified example. There is 0.5 or 50% probability of getting heads or tails. There is less probability of getting two heads in a row – 25% (0.5 × 0.5 = 0.25 or 25%). Still nothing out of the ordinary though – you would not tell your friends about it. Now if you get five heads in a row then you would take notice as the probability would be 3.1% (0.5 × 0.5 × 0.5 × 0.5 × 0.5 or $0.5^{\wedge 5}$ = 0.031 or 3.1%). Even more so with seven heads in a row as the probability is 0.78% (0.5 × 0.5 × 0.5 × 0.5 × 0.5 × 0.5 × 0.5 = 0.0078 or 0.78%). Returning to our run of data points either above or below the average, both a run of five and a run of seven have low probability of happening and so signal a likely process change if they do appear. Seven has a lower probability and so gives additional greater confidence (increases the likelihood) that a process shift has happened, and it is not just random noise. Different texts and institutions take a different stance on this tipping point in their guidance. You may wish to follow your organisation's or system's position or take a view based on the process and the likelihood of false signals. Whatever you choose, introducing this rigor will be MUCH better than relying on subjective interpretation – which is highly variable.

Other Classifications for Distinguishing Variation

In addition to considering special cause and common cause variation, another lens is to consider whether the variation is good (warranted), or bad (unwarranted).

The distinction is often contested, and the process to determine this can often take a long time – years rather than months. The NHS Atlas of Variation and the various specialism-specific NHS Getting It Right First Time reports go a long way to identifying variation and suggesting what is warranted and unwarranted. But the process of then engaging with clinicians and reducing that variation is far less proven. The gold standard example in this pursuit of unwarranted variation, with the resultant huge productivity gain, is the work of Intermountain Healthcare – an organisation we will refer to again in different sections of this book. Crucially Intermountain provide and use data on variability to empower clinicians, not to police them. Dr Terry Clemmer, then Head of ITU at Intermountain's flagship hospital in Salk Lake City, quoted by Richard Bohmer in a Harvard Business School Case Study, eloquently states "We are not trying to control the doctors. We are trying to get the doctors to control the system" (Bohmer, 2006).

John Wennberg (2002) offers a useful categorisation of unwarranted variation. His first category is **variations in effective care and patient safety**. This is where the majority of efforts to reduce unwarranted variation currently are and where the argument is perhaps clearest – often supported by clinical trial or cohort study data.

The second category is **variations in preference sensitive care**. This is where two or more effective options exist and the choice is reliant on patient preference. Wennberg notes that in reality, it is medical opinion rather than patient preference that seems to dominate the decision. This in turn creates variations in rates of procedures even across similar populations served.

The last category is **variations in supply sensitive care**. The frequency of use, by patients with chronic conditions, of things like consultations, diagnostics referrals into acute settings, hospitalisations and intensive care use is driven largely by the per capita availability to a given population. To illustrate, Wennberg states that people who live in regions with more doctors access care more. The same for regions with more beds. He states this type of variation is perplexing as medical theory, or evidence, play almost no role in this frequency of use.

Responding to Variability

Lots of organisations struggle with variation. Many take the starting point that variation is bad. Certainly, many of the points discussed in this chapter, and the perspectives discussed in Chapters 5 and 6, certainly suggest that a low variability world means you can potentially be more efficient.

As highlighted by the King's Fund (2011), paraphrasing the work of Al Mulley (The King's Fund, 2011), a common mistake is to concentrate on the outcome (the variation of outcome) rather than the process. Such as decisions to refer or not, decisions to treat or not and decisions to treat in one way or another. Like much improvement theory, it is better to concentrate on the process, and the outcomes will change – not the other way around.

Another typical response is to try and reduce variation, to try and control it with standards (sometimes called standard operating procedures, visual management, protocols or specifications). In this following section (Downham, 2016), we will discuss the use of standards, how to use appropriately to great benefit, and where their introduction can in fact make things *less* efficient.

Standards are designed to control or reduce variation. Lots of people trying to improve services, departments or teams lose sight of this. They try to standardise work for the sake of it. This is generally because they have seen the tools (standards) applied elsewhere or they view the role of management and leadership as to define the work.

The role of a standard is to limit variation in certain parts of an organisation, process or activity. They are generally focused on detailing an exercise, task or procedure to reduce variation. They are the backbone of many quality improvement initiatives as described in Chapter 2. As discussed in Chapter 3, the celebrated Keystone Project in Michigan, led by Dr Peter Pronovost, used a checklist

(Dixon-Woods, et al., 2013), form of standard, as an enabler. Although, in the face of such a tangible artefact as a checklist, it is easy to overlook the socio-cultural factors that worked in tandem with the technical to enable the huge success the project had in large-scale improvement of quality.

Appropriate reduction of variation is a good thing, but the key here is the term appropriate. In healthcare, and many social care settings, controlling *all* variation is neither appropriate nor desirable. That said, reducing variation in the *right* areas can be amazingly helpful for patients, organisations and clinicians. We want to avoid restricting those in a position to help people by wrapping them up in unnecessary standards that potentially have the unintended consequence of actually reducing our ability to help people. We will discuss this further later in this chapter.

Reducing variation can help make processes more predictable – making planning easier and helping waiting lists go down. It can help in the application of known best practice, raising confidence levels and outcomes. It can help with governance and it can improve the experience for patients.

The first step is to understand the levels of variation in a process or activity. Using techniques such as run charts and SPC charts, you can understand the nature of the variation and differentiate between natural and special cause variation. It is key to understanding whether the process or activity in question actually needs some form of activity to reduce variation in the first place.

Creating standards often makes an important contribution to the aim of controlling or reducing variation. Re-iterating an earlier point, the end point is the reduction in variation. One of the means to that end is the creation of standards. Of course, there are many other factors to consider, such as staff engagement, understanding the current levels of variation and, finally, identifying the most appropriate point for an intervention. What you want to avoid is putting in a standard to try and limit variation in human work that is in fact caused by a poor system. In this case the system would need to be redesigned, rather than a sticking plaster standard applied.

There are also lots of ways of creating and applying standards to help reduce variation. It generally depends whether you are looking at process or clinical variation. Of course, it is never that black and white as you can never tease the two fully apart – but it is useful to try to make the distinction.

Another consideration is the root cause of the variation. Lots of demands on services are in fact caused by failures in another process or activity upstream (before). You don't want to be standardising processes and activities resulting from information not being passed on, sub optimum interventions or certain information not being collected.

The words "standard", "standard operating procedure", "protocol" or "specification" don't have a great reception in healthcare. After all, healthcare is hugely complex and inherently has huge variation in much of what is demanded of it. We prefer to talk about increasing consistency of approach; something most clinicians have no problem connecting with.

It is worth considering that limiting variation is not all about paper standard operating procedures or protocols. Visual management techniques are, in many cases, intended to reduce variation around a specification. Take the most recognisable visual management standard of them all – the double yellow line. The humble double yellow line is a visual standard in the UK that is designed to standardise (reduce variation) around car parking behaviour, helping parking attendants make quick decisions around parking violations and, more importantly, help car drivers understand where they can and cannot park. Imagine what life would be like if you had to consult a book or a map to find out where you could park.

Standards are also no good if they are not upheld. It is an obvious point but one that is often under-considered. The key to ensuring standards are upheld is to make sure they are created by the people doing the work; by those who are closest to the activity and by those who have the most knowledge of the practical detail. This ideal links back to the earlier point around the move from craft to professional group-based accountability. We have worked newly integrated local authority teams who are tasked with supporting and protecting vulnerable children and have had some fantastic discussions around the role of professional accountability in upholding standards. With the teams we reflect on how it is not just about a team leader or a manager being responsible for a given standard. But rather we need to work towards the whole professional group, across disciplines, supporting and holding each other to account.

The most common form of standard in healthcare continues to be the checklist. It is not something clinicians should fear or take as a challenge to their expertise. It is simply an aid for clinicians in busy, complex and stressful situations. Situations that clinicians increasingly find themselves in.

As discussed earlier in this chapter, creating standards invariably means reducing the variety of ways that a service can respond to demand (need). If demands are standardised (patients all have the same needs) then a standardised response is efficient and effective, but on the other hand if demands are highly variable (the needs of patients vary), then a highly standardised response can be ineffective and inefficient.

Variation - Achieving the Right Balance

Depending on the presenting need, and what type of response is required, standards can be a real benefit, but they can also be undermining. Such is the complexity of health and social care, it is possible that within a single patient episode within the health service, there are places where standards are vital and some where they are counter-productive. You need to be very considered in the application of standards. They are not a blanket tool despite the flood of them being forced upon services.

Much of this flood of standardisation (sometimes referred to as specifications) is driven by:

- safety and quality thinking – a good thing
- industrial and economic theory – potentially a good thing if the work is technical, repeatable and transactional
- politics – driven by the need for accountability and rapid enforced change.

One of the dangers of standardisation (reducing variation), is defined conceptually by John Ashby in his Law of Requisite Variety (Ashby, 1956). This law states that a system must be capable of at least as much variety as the variety of the demands placed upon it – otherwise it will be overwhelmed.

He uses the sport of fencing as an example. Where if an opponent has a number of different modes of attack available, then the fencer has to have at least an equal number of modes of defence. Flipping this into healthcare system design, this means that if demands placed on a healthcare service, for example a hospital, are highly variable in type, volume and timing, then in order for the hospital to avoid being overwhelmed then the hospital has to be organised to have the capability to respond to at least that level of variability of demand.

So with hugely variable demands placed upon them, how do healthcare organisations cope? The most obvious is to standardise (restrict) entry to only certain types of work. That reduces the variety of demands, and the variation in how they present in both volume and time. This means the organisation needs to have less variety in responses available. Reduced variability in responses can lead to specialisation. This can lead to higher quality and lower cost for specific interventions. So, where variety of work demand is low, responses can be highly standardised and, in some cases, the work split into smaller, simpler tasks, standardised further and then performed by lower wage workers – a theme and consequence we will explore in depth in Chapter 8. Of course, restricting entry (referral) criteria to restrict variation and demand can just push the problem somewhere else, or delay treatment – both of which are likely to increase overall system cost.

We know that outcomes for many interventions are dependent on the healthcare determinants of health (the actions and capability of health services) and the social and environmental determinants of health. Dahlgren and Whitehead (2006), for the World Health Organisation Europe, illustrate the multiple influences, or social determinants, of a person's health as education, work environment, living and working conditions, unemployment, housing, social and community networks, individual lifestyle factors and general socio-economic, cultural and environmental conditions (Dahlgren & Whitehead, 2006). Adverse social context not only makes someone less healthy in the first place, but it also influences the way a person interacts with healthcare services. Social context introduces variability into the behaviours, responses, interactions and outcomes with healthcare services. We explore this, and the implications for quality, in depth in Chapter 11.

With this in mind, take the example of a hip replacement. The surgical inter-vention, diagnostics, procedures and referral information gathering process may be prime examples of suitable areas to work on reducing variation through stand-ardisation. Using things like decision support tools in primary care and checklists in surgical environments. Especially if the patient is perhaps "standard" in terms of clinical assessment. Hip replacements are seen as high-volume work for many providers. Extending the perspective a little, despite this standardisation and use of best practice, many systems still struggle with outcomes and end-to-end costs of such procedures. Patients get stuck in hospitals due to the lack of social care, or they arrive in hospital for their procedure not clinically fit, or they decline in wellbeing in their home environment post procedure. This is because the system is less capa-ble, in this case, of helping the person outside of the actual surgical procedure. This is because this is where the variety is often hidden – in the social and environmental determinants. In other words, in the person's life.

Returning to Ashby's law, if the whole system can cope with less variety than it is presented with, it will be overwhelmed. So, we end up with overall costs going up and patients being re-admitted or having poor post-operative outcomes. The double blow when considering this and our hip replacement example is that the same standardisation techniques that work so well in defined, bounded surgical environments have been applied, for example, to care package criteria, social care procurement and nearly all aspects of nursing. This makes them less capable of handling the variety – it stops the system doing what matters for patients – this increases costs overall.

Setting Specific Variation Considerations and Tensions

In this section we take the core principles discussed in this chapter and consider them, concisely, at the level of procedure, process and pathway, organisation and system. At each level we will also surface the variation tensions that are present and need to be at the forefront of leadership decision making. In many cases these tensions are not yet resolved, but without them being surfaced, discussed openly and kept visible, they will look like contradictions to many and serve as obstacles to improving services.

Variation at the Level of Procedure

Thinking and improvement work at this level has concentrated on procedural mode, method and timing, sequencing with other interventions (for example drug administration pre and post), communication and equipment. It is where the most work has been done on variation – for example in determining effectiveness, safety, appropriateness, preference and supply of procedures – thus allowing the distinction between warranted and unwarranted variation and the reduction of the latter. A good place to start this work is by comparing resource use by clinicians (Healthcare, 2018).

The start point is the most difficult for clinical teams looking at procedural variation. It requires investment in capable data science professionals – not just analysts but people who can work as peers with senior clinicians. A core myth to look into, and in many cases dispel, is that of "my patients are sicker than yours". The aim is to create a cycle of variation-driven enquiry. When variation occurs, there are perhaps three reasons, as Intermountain Healthcare (Healthcare, 2018) detail in their leading work on variation: 1) the patient is genuinely unique (this happens far less than is often assumed); 2) the clinician has developed a new method/knowledge/approach; or 3) there is no good reason for the variation in procedure/approach. This is a process of differentiating warranted and unwarranted variation as discussed earlier.

Of course, all of this relies on having an evidenced view on what the best practice, in terms of outcomes, efficiency and safety, actually is. It also relies on the maturity of the understanding of the use of protocols, including the baked in "override capability" (Bohmer & Edmondson, 2002) that helps to reassure clinicians. This can take decades of investment and work. That said, at the level of procedure there is widely accepted consensus on many of the procedures and interventions that make up a large proportion of the procedural work of healthcare settings.

The methods for controlling this variation at this level centre on standards, standard work packages, care bundles, reliability measurement, workplace organisation, human factors and the humble checklist.

Key tensions – tensions that leaders need to keep at the forefront:

Tension - Personalised Care vs Standardised Interventions

There is a big push for personalised care in healthcare, alongside the push to standardise the work. This is often in tension, with clinicians and leaders seeking to find the right balance between the two. In our view they do not need to be mutually exclusive. Shared decision making and patient choice can sit closely alongside exceptionally reliable and consistent procedures. The key is personalising the touch points, genuine listening, humanising the experience underpinned with high-reliability interventions.

Tension - Specification and Standardisation vs Flexibility

Another common misconception is that standardisation removes flexibility. In response, leading healthcare thinker and physician Atul Gawande argues that standardisation makes the daring possible (Gawande, 2014). Not having to worry about the reliability of core interventions and work for most patients allows clinicians to think more clearly and have time for the unusual cases that are more challenging.

The present tide of new specifications poses a slightly different challenge. Often written by those procuring services, these specifications can sometimes feel detached from the actual demands of daily work and restrict clinicians as they try to meet need. Again, the key here is in distinguishing warranted and unwarranted variation in specifications – and working with clinicians in the creation of contractual specifications in the first place.

Variation at the Level of Process and Pathway

We are in a world of interconnected multiple process steps, interventions and relationships with multiple professionals. Multiple touch points and procedures might make up a pathway or process. Variation occurs in terms of the reliability of the process or pathway (did we follow it), the outcomes and also timing and sequence. In terms of improvement theory, this is the space of QI, of process mapping and pathway improvement. Lean Thinking also dominates – with the aim being every process step shall be highly specified in content, timing and quality (Spear & Kent Bowen, 1999). In the NHS the shape of the process and pathway is often driven by tariff (payment structures) and other commissioning specifications. Tools like run charts and SPC charts help shine a light on process variation, and cumulative variation is important – that is the extent to which a pathway or process is followed. Variation in each process or pathway step is often managed through functional specialisation, the specialisation of teams or departments on a particular step/intervention, and division of labour – the division of complex tasks into smaller parts that are simpler.

Tension - Prescribed Standardisation vs High Complexity and Variability

This is where a standard, or specification, is not reflective of the work – where there has been an oversimplification of inherent variability and complexity. This puts clinicians and managers in impossible situations and is often a major factor in what may look like "resistance" to improvement initiatives. In fact, what people may be doing is drawing your attention to the complex nature of the work. Standards and specifications for high-variability processes and pathways do not have to be correspondingly complicated – simplicity (but not oversimplification) might be the key. A foundation of knowledge about the process steps where low variation really matters, and where it does not, is a strong starting point.

Tension - Pushing Standardisation vs Inherently Inefficient Processes

As discussed earlier in this chapter, standardisation is a dominant aim in many process improvement initiatives. Here at the level of process the trap is this often leads to the standardisation of either an ineffective or inefficient process. Prior to one-off, fixed standardisation, a process needs to go through an iterative prototyping phase. A phase where an improvement cycle, such as Plan, Do, Study, Act developed by Walter Shewhart (1939) and further refined by Edwards Deming (2018), is used to bring a process/pathway to a point of effectiveness and efficiency over time. This can take a large number of iterations. For example, parts of Intermountain Healthcare's celebrated Cardiovascular Pathway improvement underwent 125 iterations over four months of quality improvement (Healthcare, 2018; James & Savitz, 2011). In each iteration the process was documented into a standard that formed the basis for the next cycle. The aim was not only in reducing variation and as a result efficiency, but ensuring the process outcomes were as effective as possible before entering a period of process control. This is a stark difference to "one off" standardisation that occurs in many other settings and providers.

Tension – Flow vs Separation

There is a balance to be achieved in the urge to separate and specialise processes for flow. For example, splitting general surgery into sub-specialties (sub-groups) with their own teams and facilities. Undertaken correctly, with a process where artificial variability has been removed, separating process flows (sometimes called ring fencing) into homogenous sub-groups can be favourable in terms of efficiency, because of the opportunity to dedicate resources (Litvak & Long, 2000, p. 309). This is the same intention as the creation of value streams in Lean Thinking. In healthcare, these sub-groups and units are not necessarily existing clinical specialities, but rather sub-groups formed by the use of common resources and complementary demand (volume and arrival), variability and process variability. The key consideration in sub-dividing (separating) into sub-unit/group processes for flow is in the average flow and variability in flow in the sub-groups being considered. The tension between specialisation and standardisation is increasing efficiency at the sub-unit/group level, and the reduction in efficiency caused by reductions in utilisation[5] caused by higher flow variability as the sub-units get smaller (Litvak & Long, 2000, p. 310).

Variation at the Level of the Organisation

As the lens widens to the level of organisation, considerations turn to the management of cumulative variables and process complexity.

Consider a hospital as a V process in shape. Starting at the bottom there may be two ways of entering a hospital (urgent and non-urgent). But as options and process forks build, the number of possible iterations of process routes for a patient, and thus the management tasks, expands – the top of the V being wider than the bottom. The permeations build as departments and disciplines sub-specialise. From urgent/non-urgent at the bottom, you have medicine and surgery (two more permutations: $2 \times 2 = 4$ in total), then next up you have five to six sub-specialities

(2 × 2 × 6 = 24 permutations), 40+ sub-specialities (2 × 2 × 6 × 40 = 960 permutations), 35+ diagnostics (2 × 2 × 6 × 40 × 35 = 33600 permutations), hundreds of treatments (2 × 2 × 6 × 40 × 35 × 100 = 3.36 million permutations) and perhaps seven ways of discharging or ending the journey (2 × 2 × 6 × 40 × 35 × 100 × 7 = 23.5 million permutations) (Downham, 2016). From this simple exercise you can see how the variability of process flow and the complexity explodes – and managing such a system can become hugely difficult. The alternative to a V shaped organisation is a T shaped one. Where there is effort to reduce the discrete sub-specialisation until further downstream where personalisation takes place. This is the concept of mass customisation. The process feels personalised to the end user, but the flow happens along a few carefully designed pathways. This is similar to the concept of value streams: taking processes with hundreds of thousands of permutations but working to manage, organise, consolidate and rationalise around a handful of carefully designed sub-process groupings. The result is an organisation that is much easier to manage, but it requires the challenging of traditional professional boundaries and role definitions, as well as increasing shared resource flexibility.

As will be discussed in more detail in Chapter 5, increases in variability will always be buffered by time, capacity or inventory (Hopp & Spearman, 2000). Care needs to be taken at organisational level to notice and be aware of the increase in variability and complexity taking place within organisations. Are we always adding interventions and processes, do we ever remove some? This introduces our first tension at organisational level.

Tension - Reducing Point Cost vs Reducing Overall Process Variables (Complexity)

Take the example of a hospital considering the introduction of a diagnostic screening for an infection. Due to the point cost of the diagnostic, and variability in risk between patient groups, it would seem prudent to create a criteria for its use on incoming patients. Admitting clinicians need to follow the criteria to decide whether to run the diagnostic. This criterion might fit alongside other screening criteria. While this means the number of times the diagnostic is run can be reduced, it introduces new variation into the organisation. Clinicians need training, they need to stop and refer to the criteria, then trigger the diagnostic. There may be variability of these requests as arrival variability of patients may be high, causing issues for the lab. As we will explore further, this introduction of variability will trigger, somewhere, an increase in time, inventory (waiting patients in our case – see Chapter 5) or capacity required.

The other option is to screen everyone. This potentially adds less variability, or complexity, into the overall system of work. It is much easier to manage, to train for, as the message is easy. Over time, with economies of scale, aided by the likely reduction in arrival variability on the lab due to such high volume, the cost of the overall system end to end could well be lower than the saving of the point cost of the diagnostic.

Tension – Low In-House Variability vs Lesser Capability to Absorb Variation in Demand

The temptation, in times of pressure, is for organisations to do two things.

- The first is to run at higher levels of utilisation. As will be discussed in Chapter 5, this removal of the capacity buffer in the organisational design means the ability of the organisation to cope with arrival variation, volume variation or variation in composition (complexity) of work is greatly diminished. This will result in – some increase in inventory (patients waiting in beds), process time increase or required capacity will occur somewhere.
- The second is to tighten entry criteria. So the organisation will let in less work in the first place by reducing some types of work – reducing the variability in order to protect it, and thus the variability it needs to plan for reduces.

As discussed earlier in this chapter, Ashby's Law of Requisite Variety comes into play here. This deliberate reduction, at organisational level, in ability to cope with demand variability could mean that when such peak in variability does hit the organisation, it may not have the capability to meet the need and will become overwhelmed, either failing to cope itself or pushing work to other parts of the system in an unplanned way.

Variation at the Level of the System

Variation at the level of the system is a more established and prominent discussion in many healthcare systems. This form of variation often presents itself as variability in provision of care, resource use and outcomes.

Provision of care can often vary by geography. For example the variations in Bariatric Surgery rates across the English NHS are stark with some regions carrying out nearly double the number of procedures per 100,000 people than others. Even more challenging is that this variation generally does not match the corresponding variation in body mass index rates (GIRFT, 2017). Take another procedure, such as hip replacements, for example: the best practice in the NHS is not to use un-cemented hip replacements – but in practice this varies hugely even within regions in the English NHS, with some Health Trusts carrying out virtually zero un-cemented procedures, and others carrying them out almost exclusively – all within a relatively close geographical area (GIRFT, 2015).

Another example of variability at the system level is that of funding and corresponding availability of services. In the general practice system in the English NHS, general practices in poorer areas receive 7% less funding per need adjusted registered patient than those in less deprived areas (Fisher, et al., 2020).

Tension - Point Optimising Individual Provider Budgets vs Rising Overall Costs of Healthcare

Point optimisation is where individual departments, or organisations, optimise themselves based on their world view. This is often driven by vertically organised budget lines, management and performance measurement structures. If individual organisations optimise around their own demands, from their perspective, they point optimise and the very real danger is the system as a whole sub-optimises. This goes some way to explain why, despite relentless cost reduction exercises, overall system costs for healthcare continue to rise.

Behind this overall system cost creep is the fact point optimisation means the unmet need is passed around the system as each part of the system seeks to optimise and protect itself (generally by tightening referral criteria and scope of delivery). Each individual setting point optimises by minimising their output down to their contractual minimums and associated labelled needs. This reduces variation of what is expected of them, but this often means overall need, which is often too complex to fit within a specification, or labelled need category, is not met; perhaps due to the interplay of health and social or multi-morbidity needs. As this need is not met, then patients are in danger of increasing in need, and eventually representing somewhere else in the system at a greater level of acuity.

Conclusions

Variation is everywhere. No matter what your process, no matter what your data, all data will show variation (Poling & Wheeler, 1998, p. 85). Understanding it, considering and responding appropriately is one of the key strategies for any health system wishing to improve quality. It is clear that in many cases, using the lens of variability to question the work, the assumptions, and reduce unwarranted variability can transform interventions and vastly reduce costs. It is also clear that some variability is a good thing, and the ability of organisations to respond to variability must be baked into system and process design.

We explored in this chapter that the basic data tools exist to make better distinctions between types of variation and thus respond appropriately. John Berwick (Berwick, 1991) summarises this balance to be reached. He states:

The enemy is not considered, intentional variation, but rather unintended, or misinterpreted variation in the work of healthcare.

Levels of variability, and understanding them, must be at the centre of service design decisions. Building services with low levels of capability for handling variability for demands that have high variability will result in poor quality. Conversely, building services and processes with high levels of capability for variability but using them for demands that have low variability is high cost (Buzacott, 2000) – an obvious distinction but a trap that health services frequently fall into.

Variation continues to form a central theme in the next chapter, where we look deeply into the core challenge facing most healthcare organisations; that of managing the demands placed on them with the resources available – in other words managing demand and capacity.

Notes

1 A median (middle value in a list of numbers sorted low to high) is less influenced by outliers than an average (the term generally used to describe the arithmetic mean).
2 In some health systems wards are referred to as bed units.
3 We recommend the pragmatic texts of Donald Wheeler and Sheila Poling (Poling & Wheeler, 1998) (Wheeler, 2000).
4 Or median if using a run chart.
5 Chapter 5 features in-depth discussion on the subject of utilisation.

References

ACT Academy. 2020. *Statistical Process Control*. https://improvement.nhs.uk/documents/2171/statistical-process-control.pdf

American Society for Quality. 2020. *What Is Variation?* https://asq.org/quality-resources/variation

Ashby, R. 1956. *Introduction to Cybernetics*. Chapman & Hall / Principia Cybernetica Web.

Berwick, D.M. 1991. Controlling variation in healthcare. *Medical Care*, 29(12): 1212–1225.

Bohmer, R. 2006. *Clinical Change at Intermountain Healthcare*. Harvard Business School Publishing, N9-606-149.

Bohmer, R. and Edmondson, A. 2002. *Intermountain Healthcare*. Harvard Business School Publishing, N9-603-066.

Buzacott, J. 2000. Service system structure. *International Journal of Production Economics*, 68(1): 15–27.

Dahlgren, G. and Whitehead, M. 2006. *European Strategies for Tackling Social Inequities in Health – Levelling up Part 2*. World Health Organisation.

Deming, W. 2018. *The New Economics* (3rd edn). The MIT Press.

Dixon-Woods, M., Leslie, M., Tarrant, C. and Bion, J. 2013. Explaining Matching Michigan: An ethnographic study of a patient safety program. *Implementation Science*, 8(1): 1–13.

Downham, N. 2016. *Controlling Variation / Mass Customisation: Lean Masterclass Presentation*. Ward Downham Improvement Design Ltd.

Fisher, R., Dunn, P., Asaria, M. and Thorlby, R. 2020. *Level or Not? – Comparing General Practice in Areas of High and Low Socioeconomic Deprivation in England*. The Health Foundation.

Gawande, A. 2014. *BBC Radio 4 – The Reith Lectures*. www.bbc.co.uk/programmes/b04sv1s5

GIRFT. 2015. *Orthopaedic Surgery*. www.gettingitrightfirsttime.co.uk/surgical-speciality/orthopaedic-surgery/

GIRFT. 2017. *General Surgery*. www.gettingitrightfirsttime.co.uk/surgical-speciality/general-surgery/

Healthcare, I. 2018. *LSBU Health Services Innovation Lab Quality Improvement Study Tour* (Presentation, Salt Lake City, Utah, February 12th).

Hopp, W. and Spearman, M. 2000. *Factory Physics* (2nd edn). McGraw-Hill.

Institute of Medicine. 2001. *Crossing the Quality Chasm*. National Academies Press.

James, B.C. and Savitz, L.A. 2011. How Intermountain trimmed health care costs through robust quality improvement efforts. *Health Affairs*, 30(6): 1185–1191.

Litvak, E. and Long, M.C. 2000. Cost and quality under managed care: Irreconcilable differences? *American Journal of Managed Care*, 6(3): 305–312.

Murray, S.K., Perla, R.J. and Provost, L.P. 2011. The run chart: A simple analytical tool for learning from variation in healthcare processes. *BMJ Quality and Safety*, 20: 46–51.

Poling, S.R. and Wheeler, D.J. 1998. *Building Continual Improvement*. SPC Press.

Scholtes, P.R. 1998. *The Leader's Handbook*. McGraw-Hill.

Shewhart, W.A. 1939. *Statistical Method from the Viewpoint of Quality Control*. Department of Agriculture.

Spear, S. and Kent Bowen, H. 1999. Decoding the DNA of the Toyota Production System. *Harvard Business Review*, 77(5): 95–106.

The King's Fund. 2011. *Variations in Healthcare*. The King's Fund.

Wennberg, J. 2002. Unwarranted variations in healthcare delivery: Implications for academic medical centres. *BMJ*, 325: 961–964.

Wheeler, D.J. 2000. *Understanding Variation: The Key to Managing Chaos* (2nd edn). SPC Press.

5

Demand, Capacity and Utilisation

The Creep of High Utilisation and Its Dangers in a Variable System

Framing

In Chapter 4 we introduced and explored in depth the concept of variation - positioning it as a core quality principle including how some of the methods and classifications of variation are useful in our need to achieve a step change in quality through the deep questioning of the work of healthcare. In this chapter we will take this foundation and apply it, with an operational lens, to the common topics of organisational and process demand, capacity and utilisation. In other words, the work to be done, the resources available and the relationship between the two.

Healthcare providers have long been making improvements in quality, which again we use in a holistic sense to include not only experience, safety and equity, but also efficiency and effectiveness (Institute of Medicine, 2001). Pre-pandemic, waiting lists were shorter and processes more reliable. Despite this, in many cases services are working at their very limit - at a knife edge - and are dependent on the huge levels of discretionary effort from clinical and non-clinical staff alike. Firefighting of operational issues is commonplace, and many leaders feel there is very little extra these services can give without an injection of funding - they have reached a glass ceiling.

In this chapter we take time to set out several core operational management concepts that relate to any service. We make the case that it is a misunderstanding of these, often deceptively simple, core concepts that contributes to this glass ceiling. We look at why it is important for anyone in a leadership role to have a strong theoretical understanding of demand, capacity and the relationship between the two - which is called utilisation. We show that common misunderstandings and misconceptions in demand and capacity thinking stretch into the very top tiers of leadership. We explore how this common lack of understanding, and failure to question our assumptions and the work, is at the centre of many of the profound problems our services face - such as increasing end to end costs, stifled efforts of so-called "transformation work".

Demand - How Much Work Do We Have to Do?

Knowing how much work you, your team, your service or your organisation has to do may seem like an entirely obvious starting point, because designing a service without knowing its demand – and how that might fluctuate over time – would seem like a ludicrous way of managing. And yet, this happens all the time. In many cases the understanding of demand and the resulting capacity planning is remarkably crude. It means that problems can quickly become locked in, and a self-perpetuating cycle of firefighting of capacity issues becomes the norm. The way we build our understanding of demand strongly defines the path of improvement strategies and activities. These first steps affect all others.

Building a Systemic View of Demand

Existing demand data is often based around labelled needs (Davis, 2016). These often take the form of categories and criteria for organisational and costing purposes accompanied by codes, which we then force individual patient needs into. For example, a person with complex health and social needs has a consultation with their GP. The GP assesses their needs and then labels them so that support can be arranged. Referral documents and other similar assessment documents are used to ensure the person meets a set of criteria for each type of label and the corresponding support. This support will in turn be delivered in the form of interventions by a wide range of specialist services and/or professionals. These services have access criteria (specifications) that mean that only people with the correct label are allowed access. Each service works within its own service specifications and is performance managed based upon those specifications, and typically that service will concentrate only on the particular "need" it is funded to meet. For example, part of the role of a GP in relation to this is to fit a person's needs into labelled boxes (labelled needs) that match the range of services available. It is the structure of the services that define the boxes. The GP has to take their interpretation of need, which as we will explore in Chapter 11 can sometimes be problematic, and then describe it in a way that fits the current range and specifications of services. If the patient does not fit a labelled need, then they will not be able to get help. If they do fit a labelled need (Foundation Trust Network, 2013), that corresponding professional will invariably only concentrate on that labelled need, and only do so for as long as a pre-determined criteria is met. Note this is the design of the system, rather than the decision of the professional.

We will explore the profound impact this can have on patients later in this chapter, but in terms of building a picture of demand, what we record only represents the demand as viewed by the existing structures and services – it is a service view of demand that we have chosen to meet. This is not representative of the true demand picture as per the timing nor does it necessarily embrace the holistic nature of a person's presentation. The result is we have a picture of demand with significant blind-spots. We do not have a complete picture of the nature of the work, how much of it there is or how it varies over time. This is a very weak position to base service design and improvement decisions on.

For lack of better information, this often-flawed view will mirror the current system design, structures and response. If we genuinely want to do something different (transformational), then we need to view the work differently from the outset (Downham, 2020). This can be seen as the difference between first-order change, changes consistent with the already present schemata – the pattern of thoughts, logic and corresponding model and structure – and second order change, changes to the schemata itself (Bartunek & Moch, 1987). If we are seeking transformational improvement, then understanding the fundamental nature and variability of demand (need) as early as possible, before it has been distorted by labels and process, is an essential step in order to innovate and transform.

This step of fundamentally understanding demand has parallels with Lean Thinking. The first of five Lean principles that form the basis of the famous codification of the hugely successful Toyota Production System by Jones and Womack (2003) is Understanding Value. This is a deliberate step to take time to understand what is the value proposition which the entire organisation should be centred on delivering. This is a radical step because it moves an organisation away from delivering what is efficient, assumed or convenient, to one that focuses on delivering value, in our case meeting need, as quickly and reliably as possible.

This is better described in relation to service industries, like healthcare, as Understanding Purpose (Bicheno, 2012, p. 11). Purpose is often not at all clear in healthcare – with a clinician often in the middle of competing and impossible tensions between their personal views, views of management, views of peers, the wishes of patients and the wishes of those who govern and commission services. The ultimate illustration of this is a patient deciding not to have further interventions at the end of life – despite the awesome capability of medical science to prolong life. This may be contrary to the view of some professionals, and even sometimes the views of members of the patient's family, but a good and peaceful death is what represents value to them.

Variation in Demand

Consider a typical health service. A common approach to planning would be to consider the average demand per week. A figure that has been derived by looking at historic demand (as illustrated in Figure 5.1). Let's assume the service has gone some way to avoid the traps discussed previously in this chapter by using the referrals received per week rather than a figure of procedures per week actually completed (which would invariably be a product of capacity). For this service the average referral demand per week is 150 procedures. The service is then staffed on this number (after converting the procedures to hours).

Perhaps there is a degree of confidence in the figure of 150, as the year before that produced similar. So all is good? Perhaps not – let's explore why this is problematic.

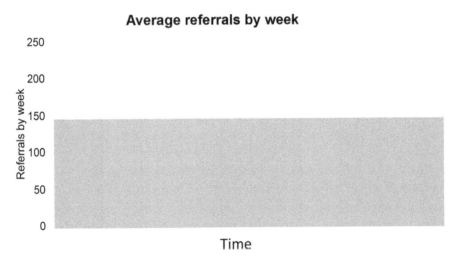

Figure 5.1   Average demand

The Impact of Variability on Operational Management

The dataset that this average figure was derived from can be found in Figure 5.2. It shows the previous year's demand varying around its average. The average figure from Figure 5.1 can be seen as the horizontal dashed line.

When looking at Figure 5.2, we can see that this data is far more useful than the average figure of 150. This is the power of a graphical representation of data. Plotting that data over time, in the form of a run chart, allows the visualisation of the variability – see the solid line in Figure 5.2.

As we discussed in Chapter 4, a run chart is the graphical display of data plotted in some form of order (Murray et al., 2011), in this case in time interval order. The number of referrals per week is represented by the vertical Y axis and the weekly time interval is plotted on the horizontal X axis. Considering ourselves as the manager, the fact the time interval of the plot is in weeks provides us with much greater clarity than if it was represented by a monthly figure, or even quarterly figure – the two latter intervals masking much of the actual demand variation at play. Plotting data over time, regardless of whether it is demand data or, for example, safety or process capability data, is useful because it provides context to interpret the data (Wheeler, 2000). The fact you can see the variation from data point to data point and over a broader time period allows for a more informed interpretation.

In Figure 5.2 you can also see that the demand fluctuates from week to week – it shows variability – it is variation. It is these variations that are important to understand. As the manager in this service, would you rather plan using the average figure? Or plan using the knowledge of how the referral demand varied by week – the variation?

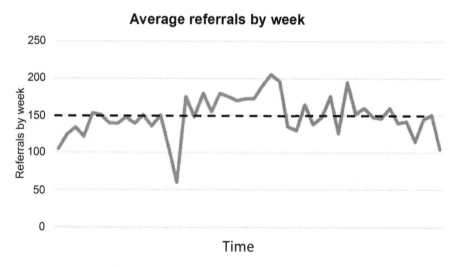

Figure 5.2   Variability of demand

A manager would undoubtedly want to understand the variation of demand, rather than have the average figure. How the demand varies by week, understanding the full range of peaks and troughs, and making a judgement based on the patterns of the demand variation enables the manager to make more accurate judgements regarding how to plan their service in order to respond. If the manager had planned their service to meet the average demand, they would have been caught out with excess demand a considerable proportion of the time.

If the demand was static, as an average figure suggests, if there was no variability, then services would be very easy to plan (Litvak & Long, 2000) and our health and social care services would run like clockwork. Staffing could be arranged, facilities organised, financials certain and consumables ordered in confidence. Downstream processes (things that come after our intervention) would be able to plan on this certainty and there would be fewer peaks and troughs of work. It is variability that hits productivity and makes teams, departments, organisations and systems so difficult to manage. If the work was always the same and it arrived at standard intervals then things would be straightforward. Taiichi Ohno, the engineer credited with creating the Toyota Production System,[1] labelled this form of variation as inconsistency (unevenness) or *mura* (Ohno, 1988, p. 41). Much of his work was dedicated in removing unevenness from demand profiles and other areas of variation within processes; in other words, making them more predictable. Hopp and Spearman also focus attention on the role variation plays in the throughput and outcomes organisations aim for. They detail two *laws*:

1. Law (Variability): Increasing variability always degrades performance of a production system.
2. Law (Variability Buffering): Variability in a production system will be buffered by some combination of:
   - Inventory
   - Capacity
   - Time

(Hopp & Spearman, 2000, p. 295)

The language here is strong, and obviously originates from the manufacturing sector, but the message is still applicable and clear. There will be consequences if variability is increased. If variability is increased, whether that is a new member of staff, a new additional diagnostic option, changes to referral criteria, change in patient volumes, new staff, changes to staffing patterns or changes to referral patterns – to name just a few – there will be consequences to the overall process and system of work. If this is done in a considered way, such as new staff are introduced knowing that the overall system throughput will decrease for a period of time, and that is planned for appropriately, then that might be an acceptable trade-off. But if this is done in an uncontrolled manner – such as the changing of a supplier or changing of a rota without the other interconnected parts of the system being informed – then there will be a consequence to this increase in variability. Contextualising for healthcare, they suggest variability has three consequences. High variability will either lead to one or a combination of the following:

Variability Buffered with Inventory

In the most literal sense, when considering something like an equipment or consumable supply chain, this would mean increased inventory levels at various points of the supply chain in order to buffer variability. This means holding inventory to cope with fluctuations, on either the demand or supply side of the supply chain. Inventory costs money to hold. Regardless of whether inventory, for example in a hospital, is held on consignment (owned by the supplier until use), the cost of that inventory is still borne by the supply chain – so the cost will be built into the pricing. Variation in consumable supply chains will raise prices and it is in the best interest of the hospital, in the case of our example, and the supplier to reduce it.

In terms of impact on our broad definition of quality, including effectiveness and efficiency, the other type of inventory that hospitals hold dwarfs that of consumables and equipment. This is the inventory of patients, held in wards. Patients in a ward can be split into two types:

1) Those in a bed awaiting an assessment, decision, intervention or diagnostic of some kind of trigger/signal for them to move forward in their care
2) Those in a bed for genuine care reasons (is it the best place for them right now?) and cannot be moved forward by any additional assessment, decision, intervention or diagnostic (other than for monitoring of wellbeing and progression of previous interventions)

Patients of the first type are like inventory. They are a consequence of the system and a buffer for variability. A buffer for either decision-making variability, the availability of the right person or information to make a decision on them – or downstream capacity variation such as social care capacity in the community, or capacity variation for an intervention. They are being held, or in other words warehoused, due to the variability in the wider hospital system. The costs of all these buffering patients in beds is substantial, with the unit cost of an excess bed day being £346.00/day (NHS Improvement, 2018).

Variability Buffered with Capacity

The second form of variability buffer is extra capacity. Variability in demand, in terms of volumes and arrival frequency, can result in the need for extra capacity – to absorb the peaks in demand or to minimise the troughs in capacity. This could be in the form of equipment or facilities capacity such as operating theatres, or it could be in the form of workforce. If, for example, demand did not vary then staff could be organised in a much more cost-effective manner. Overtime and extra shifts could be avoided.

Variability Buffered with Time

The third form of variability buffer is time. This could be in one or a combination of waiting time, end-to-end time and/or procedure time. With no other counter-measure in place, an increase in variability will result in an increase in time – which invariably translates to waiting time. Things take longer.

The Practical Reality

When considering these three forms of variability buffer (consequences of variability), health services rely on inventory and time most commonly. Increasing time does not increase either variable or the fixed costs in the short term. Bed stock is a fixed cost and bed levels, regardless of whether they are full of "inventory" patients or not, are relatively static.[2] Wards, as units of care, can only be opened in a stepped rather than gradual fashion due to the practical minimum staffing and size of typical wards – thus making them difficult, and very financially noticeable, in their flexible use as a tool to buffer variability other than for seasonal variability such as opening an extra ward for winter flu pressures. Long term though, this does go some way to explaining why such large numbers of beds are required. They buffer the variability of the system.

This leaves time as the most common form of variability buffer. The waiting times experienced in many healthcare systems are, to a significant extent,[3] a direct buffer to the inherent variability in all parts of the system. This could be seen in a delay in getting an appointment in general practice, long waits for surgical procedures or even waiting lists to register for NHS dentists.

Stepping back a little here, the important thing is to consider these as working principles – to ensure consideration of variability is front and centre in a leader's mind.

Continuing our theme of understanding demand, there are a huge number of sources of variation. Some of them are influenced by the customer (or patient) in the form of arrival, requests, capability, effort and subjective preference (Frei, 2006). Other sources in the form of arrival variation can come from upstream process variation, such as the variations in referral from a general practice into surgical specialists or in the transfer of patients from one department to another in a hospital. Treatment and decision making in healthcare can often vary from known best practice in terms of effectiveness and patient safety. Resource use also varies and is driven by preference, although the choice of the patient is often driven by the clinician and supply – the available supply of healthcare drives resource use (Wennberg, 2002). An example of this is the work of Rebecca Rosen of the Nuffield Trust, cited in Walley et al. (2019). Rosen found that 19% of patients using primary care walk in clinics in the NHS *would have not bothered to seek care if this service had not been available* (Rosen, 2014).

All of these things drive demand variability for downstream processes and so can lead to costly buffering.

Capacity - How Much Work Can We Do?

Our ability to do different types of work in healthcare systems varies by day, week, month and year for many of the reasons discussed in the previous section on demand. While teams, departments and organisations generally have a better understanding of their capacity, because it is so closely financially monitored, there are still a number of important, but often overlooked, points that need to be considered when planning capacity in relation to demand. We will briefly summarise them here and bring them to life in terms of implications later in this chapter.

Variability

Capacity varies in the same way demand does. The ability of a team, service or organisation to do work is hugely variable, and is not just a product of the number of staff or availability of physical capacity such as operating theatre capacity. Sources of variability include the holiday and training patterns, skill mix, start and finish times, and morale of staff, as well as countless detractors from the core job, such as meetings, calls and emails, equipment, IT issues and facilities problems. The impact of this can be substantial. In studies on nurse direct care time, as little as 37% of a nurse's time is spent directly caring for patients – either physically or undertaking psycho-social care (NHS Institute for Innovation and Improvement, 2008). This is likely to be an over-estimate as this starts from a point of the nurse being on the ward at the start of the shift. There are significant additional losses and variability in capacity caused by holidays, rota patterns, training, sickness and absence. To this point a study of community nursing found that taking this macro level starting point found that direct care time was just 21% of total contracted hours (NHS Institute for Innovation and Improvement, 2010).

The compounding factor in these figures, and countless other examples of capacity losses, is their variability over time. These losses vary by minute, hour, day, week, month and year. They "spike" pathways and cause surge or famine fluctuations in the work downstream and bottlenecks upstream. This capacity variation is one of the reasons it is so hard to have high reliability in process outcomes in large healthcare providers.

Earlier in this chapter, we discussed Hopp and Spearman's variability laws in relation to demand. Those laws also apply in terms of detailing why certain levels of capacity are required and, as such, are an important rule of thumb for any manager.

Decision-Making Capability

Every decision every...

One of the biggest drivers of our ability to do work (our capacity), and make things flow in healthcare is decision-making capability. The thing that drives our complex healthcare processes is the ability to make the right decision, promptly, in order to trigger the next onward step. If this capability does not exist then patients end up queuing (often buffered in beds on wards) waiting for the decision on an onward step. As discussed, this waiting is completely different to legitimate recovery and care time, and is often completely avoidable. In one of the most formative experiences of our time in healthcare, in a quick audit of patients in wards in a regional hospital we found that one-third of all patients were waiting for decisions to be made in order for them to move forward in their journey ("inventory" patients – using our previous categorisation).

Manufacturing organisations, especially those adopting Lean Thinking, have been aware for a long time of the issues of batching up work. They drive for the smallest batch sizes possible as this reduces costly work in process and also reduces lead times. A measure of this often used is the "Every Product Every" Interval. Manufacturing plants use this measure to steadily drive down batch sizes so they can make every product every month, to every week, to every day. Each decrease in batch sizing takes out huge chunks of costly work in process (inventory) from the balance sheet.

The problem of work in process and of batch sizing is equally applicable to healthcare, and far beyond the obvious transferability to operating theatres. In healthcare, as described previously, work in process, inventory, is very often people in beds. Batching directly translates to batching of decisions. If decisions on patients are batched up, for example for a weekly MDT, ward round or a particular consultant's availability, then patients will stack up waiting as inventory / work in process. This inventory of patients is acting as a buffer to poor process in a similar way to that described in Hopp and Spearman's (2000) Variability Laws explored earlier in this chapter. You could describe some wards in hospitals that are struggling with this as warehouses of people waiting for decisions to be made on them. In other words, as former Chief Economist for the American Commerce Department's Office of Policy Development Lee Price stated in the *Economist*, "Inventory (in our case people in beds) is a substitute for information" (Price, 2000). Make decisions at shorter intervals, and hospitals and other healthcare services flow better. Figure 5.3 illustrates how reducing decision-making batches (increasing decision-making flexibility) directly impacts length of stay.

The X axis is the frequency of decisions a hospital, for example, is capable of, and the Y axis is the number of patients waiting for decisions (work in process – often in beds, blocking other work, having a poor experience and costing money). The grey line illustrates the growing number of patients waiting for a decision in a hospital that only has the capability it needs to make *every decision every* week. The horizontal grey dashed line illustrates the average number of patients waiting. The black line illustrates a hospital with the capability to make *every decision every day*. The horizontal dashed black line illustrates the average number of patients waiting – one seventh of the number of the hospital with poorer decision-making flexibility. Of course, we know that a lot goes into a decision in healthcare. It is a product of a person(s) with the requisite skillset, the right diagnostic information and access to the correct and joined up patient records – it is also increasingly made in partnership with the patient. Given the impact it has, there is a real imperative for healthcare organisations to question traditional decision-making practices in order to improve information flow. They should strive to support and enable decision making at the safest lowest level and thus increase the frequency decisions can be made at. This is referred to as maximum subsidiarity and something we will refer to in Chapter 9. This can be achieved by investing in decision-making frameworks and repositioning expertise to the role of supporting and enabling the reliable delivery of world-class decisions, rather than making them. MDT meetings can be made more frequent through better preparation and the use of information technology.

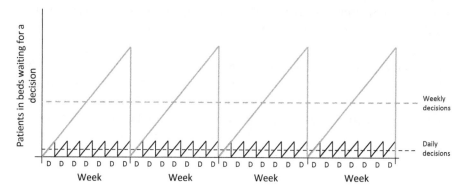

Figure 5.3   Decision making

Utilisation - The Fractious Relationship between Demand and Capacity

Utilisation (Ut) is a figure derived from dividing demand by capacity – see Figure 5.4. It gives a percentage of the proportion of capacity that is taken up in order to meet demand. 50% Ut means that half of our capacity is used meeting demand; 100% Ut means all of our capacity is used in meeting demand. This Ut figure is hugely useful in understanding the fluctuating relationship between demand (the work you need to do) and capacity (the work you can do).

$$Ut = \frac{\text{Demand}}{\text{Capacity}}$$

Figure 5.4   Utilisation equation (Bicheno, 2012; Kingman, 1961)

This relationship is at the core of managing any team, service or organisation. When capacity is bigger than demand, then all is well, a service can meet its commitments – this feels like a good day. When demand is bigger than capacity, a team cannot meet its commitments. With all the performance and patient pressure this entails, it will feel like a difficult day. In short, many front line staff, and their leaders, live and breathe the consequences of utilisation levels every day. As we will explore in this chapter, the level of utilisation is not only the key for unlocking delays and flow, but also the key to staff wellbeing and patient safety.

Sweating the Asset – Utilisation in Action and Compounding Factors

Imagine a time when a service had more than enough capacity to meet its demand. In other words, utilisation is low. The run charts in Figure 5.5 illustrate this. The X axis details time intervals, and the Y axis details a common unit for both capacity and demand (hours). The grey line details the demand, and how it is varying over time. The black line details capacity, and how that is also varying over time. In this case the black capacity line is consistently above the grey demand line. The two lines never intersect, and we have what is known as "headroom". Because capacity is bigger than demand our utilisation figure is less than 100%. In this case it is 64%.

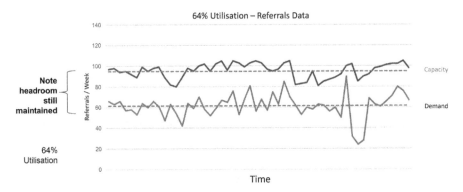

Figure 5.5   Low utilisation

Because in this case, capacity is bigger than demand, queues will always be low. If there is a peak demand point that coincides with low capacity, then subsequent days will recover the situation. In other words, due to the low utilisation, the headroom, the service can dig itself out of any problems it finds itself in.

Now low utilisation is often regarded as a dirty term. It has connotations of not being productive and not "sweating the asset". From a traditional Western management point of view, the drive would be to increase utilisation of a service. After all, you want it doing the most work possible don't you? Figure 5.6 shows the impact of increasing the utilisation slightly. In this case raising it to 78%. You can see here that as the utilisation has increased, the black capacity line and the grey demand line have moved closer together. The key to this is the variability of both lines. You can see from the first half that the lines never intersected, so a queue would not have built, but later in the timeline, they did begin to intersect and a queue would have built. This is despite the averages for both being different and there being headroom between them. It is all about the variation around the average. Depending on the timing of the demand and capacity variability, the service might be lucky and no queue build, or they might not, potentially surging or starving downstream processes. Is luck a basis for managing services?

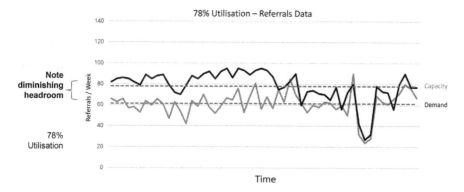

Figure 5.6 Increasing utilisation

The temptation to increase utilisation is always there though. Perhaps the service has a cost improvement plan to meet, and so reduces capacity – thus increasing utilisation. *But this will be ok if we ensure demand and capacity is balanced… right?* The answer is no.

Figure 5.7 shows the service at 100% utilisation. Demand and capacity are balanced. At this point a queue will begin to form as the demand and capacity lines vary and begin to overlap. Even though they have the same average, a queue and resulting wait can and will build.

The failure to grasp this is something services find very difficult to shake. The ill-advised drive to balance demand and capacity is even prevalent in improvement guidance from thought leaders (The Health Foundation, 2013; Healthcare Improvement Scotland, 2021), central NHS improvement training programmes (NHS Improvement, 2017) and in statements we hear on a regular basis from clinical and non-clinical leaders in both primary and secondary care. You cannot run a service at 100% utilisation, with demand and capacity balanced, and not have

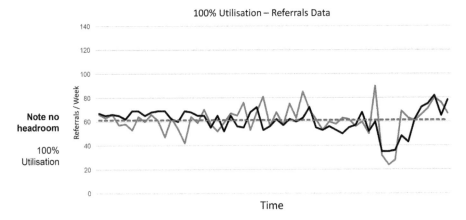

Figure 5.7 100% utilisation

delays and waits build. In fact, as utilisation increases, delays will increase in a highly non-linear fashion (Hopp & Spearman, 2000, p. 303).

Figure 5.8 shows our previous three levels of utilisation and the impact on waits. Note the non-linear fashion of the delay increase. Things get out of control quickly when utilisation approaches 100%. The higher the levels of inherent variability in the processes (demand, capacity, arrival and process variability (Kingman, 1961)), the lower the levels of utilisation that trigger sharp increases in waits and unpredictability. If we consider the huge levels of inherent variability in healthcare processes, it is safe to assume that low levels of utilisation are required in order to avoid chaotic increases in delays and unpredictability.

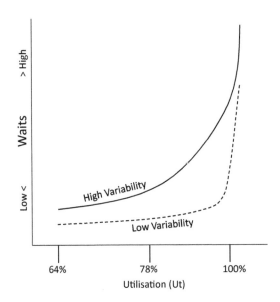

Figure 5.8 Relationship between Ut and waits (Adapted from Bicheno, 2012)

Despite this, taking the NHS as an example, its levels of bed utilisation are regularly run at 90% as illustrated in Figure 5.9, leaving very little headroom in a highly variable system – triggering all the consequences we have discussed. It is worth noting that it is this unpredictability that is most damaging as it means services cannot promise or plan with any reliability.

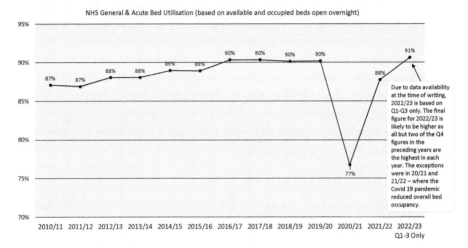

NHS General & Acute Bed Utilisation (based on available and occupied beds open overnight)

Figure 5.9 NHS England bed utilisation (source data from NHS England, n.d.)

So why is it that waits and queues always build with high utilisation? Why can we not match demand and capacity? This is the second of the great, institutionalised misunderstandings seen in the planning of services in healthcare. Demand and capacity do not behave in the same way – they are fundamentally different. Capacity is lost if not used. It cannot be stored up for the next day. Demand can be stored up. Generally, in healthcare settings if demand is not met, due to variation in capacity or greater than expected arrival (variation in demand), then it will still be there the next day. This compounding nature of demand is the difference. This is why demand and capacity cannot be matched without severe consequences. To cater for this compounding nature of demand, capacity needs to be higher than demand (lower utilisation) in order for delays and unpredictability not to build.

So What Should the Level of Utilisation Be?

There are a number of rules of thumb thrown around that are not particularly helpful in answering this question – such as 80%. The true answer is "it depends". It depends on the inherent variability of the process in question. Figure 5.8, referred to previously, also shows two scenarios. One with high inherent variability in the process and one with lower variability. The process with low variability, illustrated with the dashed line, can run at higher levels of utilisation before delays and unpredictability increase sharply. This is obviously extremely attractive to service managers under throughput pressure and finance managers wishing to "sweat the asset". The reason for this is shown in Figure 5.10.

Graph A in Figure 5.10 illustrates a process with high variability. In this case its demand (black line) and its capacity (grey line) are highly variable. The implication of this is you cannot bring the two lines together (increase utilisation) very closely before the lines intersect at some point and queues and unpredictability increase. Graph B in Figure 5.10 illustrates a process with lower variability. The demand and the capacity lines are not going up and down so much, they have less variation. It is possible in this scenario to bring the two lines much closer and increase utilisation to a much higher extent before the lines begin to intersect and queues and unpredictability increase. So with low variability a service can have its cake (high utilisation) and eat it too (low queues and less chaos).

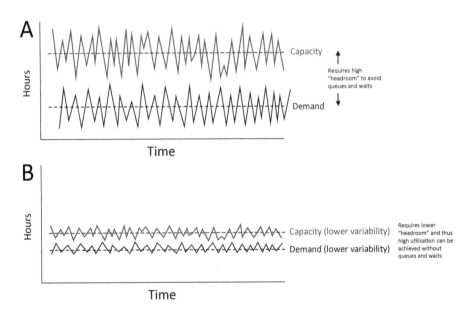

Figure 5.10   Reducing variability to increase utilisation

The answer to the question about *what level of utilisation is required?* is whatever the level of variability allows. If the process is highly variable then utilisation needs to be low, otherwise the variability will be buffered through a wait, but if there is low variability then it can operate at high utilisation. It is process specific. A great place to start is to create specific demand and capacity run charts for the process or service in order to begin to understand the inherent variability in it. Then consideration can be given to how close the lines can be brought together before the headroom disappears – a judgement that is specific to the process and the specific variability within it.

Aggravating Factors

As if the above situation was not bad enough, with the levels of unpredictability and delays exponentially increasing as services seek to increase utilisation, sweat the asset and attempt to dig themselves out of issues by working the system harder, there are two further issues that aggravate the situation and often bring the system and staff to breaking point:

- Rewarding
- Pressurising

The first is that systems of reward and performance managing individuals and teams just exacerbate the problem. Due to the inherent variability in typical processes, a good "performance" or bad "performance" is often down to the process variation – in this case whether the peaks and troughs of demand and capacity overlap. This is about the process, not the individuals within it. If staff are pressurised (performance managed or even ranked) due to this process variation, something which is not in their control, then it serves to further demotivate them. After all, it is the managers and leaders who own the process that front line staff work within. This is explored in depth in the summary lessons from Deming's famous Red Bead exercise – illustrating the futility of many reactive management actions and performance management decisions (Deming, 2018, p. 117).

Reactive Extra Capacity

The second aggravating factor is based on a further process law from Hopp and Spearman.

Law (Capacity): In steady state (in the long run), all plants (organisations / processes) will release work at an average rate that is strictly less than the average capacity.

(Adapted from Hopp & Spearman, 2000, p. 303)

This is due to the variability in the capacity of interconnected process steps. Sooner or later, those peaks and troughs have the effect of starving downstream processes and causing bottlenecks in front of upstream processes. It may take time, but eventually this always results in outputs being less than the average capacity (Goldratt, 1990; Hopp & Spearman, 2000), because, as previously stated, capacity is lost in time if not used.

Using the example of surgery in a hospital, the failure to grasp this results in repeated cycles of extra lists and other waiting list initiatives when backlogs inevitably appear; backlogs that are due to running at too high a level of utilisation than the current levels of variability will allow for, and also by mistakenly planning outputs to be in line with average capacity. These backlogs result in increases in waiting time for patients and also slippages in length of stay – as all processes within a pathway (imaging, wards, pre-assessment etc.) begin to operate at levels of high utilisation which are beyond what the current levels of variation will tolerate. Eventually this mess shows up on the hospital performance metrics and pressure from leaders is applied to staff (note this is a process issue not a staff issue). A one-off waiting list initiative is then authorised, and extra lists are planned. This increases capacity dramatically and thus reduces utilisation. The delays and backlogs reduce. Those with influence over the process (leaders) then fail to reflect upon the systemic causes of the original issue, and under pressure to cut the costs of the extra lists now the process delay is under control, take out the extra capacity and return the process to its original steady state. The expectation is that the output will be the average capacity of the process and also that the process should run at a level of utilisation that cannot be tolerated with the current levels of process variation. Inevitably, sooner or later, the natural peaks and troughs land unfavourably, and the cycle begins again. Hopp and Spearman call this the Overtime Vicious Cycle.

Death Spiral

Finally, it is important to consider the eventual human cost of high utilisation and misguided pressuring of staff. High levels of utilisation put teams under huge pressure. It is where individuals resort to using their discretionary effort, such as not breaking for lunch or even to go to the toilet, on list overruns and working in the evenings, in order to keep pace with work demands. It is worth stating that in healthcare services there is a huge reliance on this discretionary effort to make the capacity side of the utilisation equation bigger and thus reduce utilisation. This reliance on discretionary effort, especially over a prolonged period of time, can tip a team into a figurative *death spiral*. This is because individuals and teams working flat out increases stress. In the end the stress and exhaustion take their toll and eventually a team member may go off sick. This reduces the capacity in our utilisation equation and increases utilisation and thus the burden on those remaining. This stress takes its toll again and eventually another team member goes off sick. This in turn increases utilisation and so on… a death spiral where a team struggles to even achieve minimum of staff levels reliably and is often reliant on agency staff or has high levels of staff turnover of vacancies. All of which contribute to lower levels of effective capacity and increased utilisation.

Conclusions

In this chapter we have explored the core concept of utilisation. While seemingly abstract in the form of an equation, the dynamic between demand and capacity, the work arriving and the amount of work that can be done, is absolutely the core of quality challenges facing healthcare teams, organisations and systems.

Through this discussion we learned that high levels of utilisation, in systems of work with high variability, will ALWAYS result in queues and confusion. We also learned that the classic responses of things like waiting list efforts are not effective as they don't address the fundamental issue of the variability of capacity and variability of demand. The conclusion here is the need to examine and question the planning of teams and organisations using the principles of utilisation and variation.

In the next chapter we continue with the utilisation equation but question it. We show how you can reduce utilisation by employing effective strategies – strategies that don't require extra capacity. The core of this being the reduction of detractors to capacity, and the reduction of demands based on failures in the system – Failure Demand.

Acknowledgements

We would like to thank John Bicheno for his writing and teaching that has triggered much of the thinking in this chapter.

Notes

1 This system was the foundation for Toyota to grow from obscurity into the world's leading car maker. As of 2020 it continues to be the most valuable car making brand (Statista, 2020).
2 Although over a longer time window, bed stock in most healthcare systems has been reducing.
3 The other main reason is over-utilisation, which is explored later in this chapter.

References

Bartunek, J. and Moch, M. 1987. First-order, second-order and third-order change and organisational development interventions: A cognitive approach. *JABS Classic Papers*, 23(4): 483–500.

Bicheno, J. 2012. *The Service Systems Toolbox*. Picsie Books.

Davis, R. 2016. *Responsibility in Public Services*. Triarchy Press.

Deming, W. 2018. *The New Economics* (3rd edn). The MIT Press.

Downham, N. 2020. *Understanding the Work of Healthcare*. www.cressbrookltd.co.uk

Foundation Trust Network. 2013. *FTN Benchmarking Operating Theatres*. https://nhsproviders.org/media/1148/ftnb-ot-case-study-avoiding-last-minute-cancellations.pdf

Frei, F. 2006. Breaking the trade-off between efficiency and service. *Harvard Business Review*, 84(11): 93–101.

Goldratt, E. 1990. *Theory of Constraints*. The North River Press Publishing Corporation.

Healthcare Improvement Scotland. 2021. *Access QI – Maximising Service Capacity and Capability*. https://ihub.scot/project-toolkits/access-qi-covid-19-maximising-service-capacity-and-capability/maximising-service-capacity-and-capability-change-package/stage-4-implementing-and-refining-changes/balancing-demand-and-capacity/

Hopp, W. and Spearman, M. 2000. *Factory Physics* (2nd edn). McGraw-Hill.

Institute of Medicine. 2001. *Crossing the Quality Chasm*. National Academies Press.

Jones, D. and Womack, J. 2003. *Lean Thinking* (1st edn). Simon & Schuster UK Ltd.

Kingman, J. 1961. The single server queue in heavy traffic. *Mathematical Proceedings of the Cambridge Philosophical Society*, 57(4): 902–904.

Litvak, E. and Long, M.C. 2000. Cost and quality under managed care: Irreconcilable differences? *American Journal of Managed Care*, 6(3): 305–312.

Murray, S.K., Perla, R.J. and Provost, L.P. 2011. The run chart: A simple analytical tool for learning from variation in healthcare processes. *BMJ Quality and Safety*, 20: 46–51.

NHS England. n.d. *Bed Availability and Occupancy Data – Overnight*. www.england.nhs.uk/statistics/statistical-work-areas/bed-availability-and-occupancy/bed-data-overnight/

NHS Improvement. 2017. *ACT Academy*. www.england.nhs.uk/wp-content/uploads/2020/08/QSIR-A5–4pp.pdf

NHS Improvement. 2018. *Reference Costs 2017/18: Highlights, Analysis and Introduction to the Data*. https://improvement.nhs.uk/documents/1972/1_-_Reference_costs_201718.pdf

NHS Institute for Innovation and Improvement. 2008. *Releasing Time to Care: The Productive Ward – Executive Leader's Guide*. NHS Institute for Innovation and Improvement.

NHS Institute for Innovation and Improvement. 2010. *Productive Community Services: Releasing Time to Care – Managing Caseload and Staffing*. NHS Institute for Innovation and Improvement.

Ohno, T. 1988. *Toyota Production System – Beyond Large-Scale Production*. Taylor and Francis.

Price, L. 2000. Enter the eco-system – from supply chain to network. *The Economist*, 11 November.

Rosen, R. 2014. *Meeting Need or Fuelling Demand: Improved Access to Primary Care and Supply-Induced Demand*. The Nuffield Trust.

Statista, 2020. *Most Valuable Brands within the Automotive Sector as of 2020, by Brand Value.* www.statista.com/statistics/267830/brand-values-of-the-top-10-most-valuable-car-brands/

The Health Foundation. 2013. *Improving Patient Flow across Organisations and Pathways.* www.health.org.uk/sites/default/files/ImprovingPatientFlowAcrossPathways AndOrganisations.pdf

Walley, P., Found, P. and Williams, S. 2019. Failure Demand: A concept evaluation in UK primary care. *International Journal of Health Care Quality Assurance*, 32(1): 21–33.

Wennberg, J. 2002. Unwarranted variations in healthcare delivery: Implications for academic medical centres. *BMJ*, 325: 961–964.

Wheeler, D.J. 2000. *Understanding Variation: The Key to Managing Chaos* (2nd edn). SPC Press.

6

Understanding Failure Demand

Capacity Detractors, Failure Demand and Reducing Utilisation

Framing

In Chapter 5 we introduced the concept of utilisation and its relevance to the daily and strategic operations management of most healthcare providers, regardless of role, shape or form. We learnt how high levels of utilisation in highly variable settings set off a compounding chain of events, creating queues like a snowball rolling down a hill getting bigger and bigger. Chapter 5 also determined that the tactics of working harder or sporadic increases in capacity in order to reduce utilisation are not effective long term. So, what other strategies are there?

The utilisation equation provides a useful starting point (Figure 6.1). The equation shows that to reduce utilisation either demand needs to be reduced or capacity increased. As discussed in Chapter 5, the prudent approach is to understand and reduce the variability within both.

$$Ut = \frac{Demand}{Capacity}$$

Figure 6.1 Utilisation equation (Bicheno, 2012)

In this chapter we explore the strategies for both in detail. In doing so we will introduce and explore the concept and strategies for the reduction of capacity detractors. We will then move on to introduce the concept of Failure Demand – which we define as avoidable demand that is of our own making. Finally, we conclude this chapter by presenting a framework of four domains from which avoidable Failure Demand can be seen to arise – the systemic sources of Failure Demand. We argue that these domains need to be well understood if we are to break the glass ceiling of quality in services.

Reducing Capacity Detractors

Starting the capacity side, there is a need to understand where the losses in capacity are coming from. These losses can be described as detractors (Hopp & Spearman, 2000), as they detract from base capacity – as illustrated in Figure 6.2; reduce capacity detractors and capacity increases.

$$Ut = \frac{Demand}{Base\ Capacity - Detractors}$$

Figure 6.2   Capacity detractors

In health services there is a lot of emphasis on increasing capacity. It is often the first request to ask for more staff. In many health systems there have been periods of huge growth in healthcare funding, although some years in the past now, much of which was focused on increasing capacity. For example, in the UK under the then Labour government's NHS spending pledge, funding increased 7% between 2000/2001 and 2010/2011 (The King's Fund, n.d.). But there is less appetite to "buy our way" out of trouble in the present day and a strong argument that unfocused extra capacity (or supply) can simply increase healthcare usage rather than improve outcomes (Berwick, 2008; Wennberg, 2002).

Because of the lack of availability of extra funding, getting the most out of present capacity is often the focus of quality improvement initiatives. Many of which are focused on capacity detractors which result in the capacity losses we discussed in the previous chapter – such as the fact that as little as 37% of a nurse's time is spent directly caring for patients – either physically or undertaking psycho-social care (NHS Institute for Innovation and Improvement, 2008). The quality improvement tools often used are:

- **Set up reduction**. This originates from the teachings of Shigeo Shingo's Single Minute Exchange of Die (SMED) system (Shingo, 1985) and is widely used to reduce the variability and overall set-up and change-over times in settings such as operating theatres.
- **Workplace organisation**. Often using the 5S methodology (Hirano, 1995), this is the physical organisation of the workplace in order to reduce staff time losses

(detractors) and mistakes, the application of which is widely seen in most health-care settings from wards and operating theatres, to pharmacy, imaging and so on.

- **Time study**. With a lineage dating back to the work of F.W. Taylor (2005) and Frank and Lillian Gilbreth (1910–1919) this is the deep study of workers and how they go about their work. In the English NHS, this method was popularised through the introduction of the Activity Follow technique in the nationally adopted Productive Series of quality improvement programmes that is explored in detail in Chapter 2 (NHS Institute for Innovation and Improvement, 2008).

- **Error proofing**. Again, originating from the work of Shigeo Shingo (1987), error proofing is the process of removing the possibility of mistakes from processes, moving from reliance on audit and compliance, to making it impossible for something to be "done wrong". Common applications are in valve fittings, equipment assembly and in user interface design in electronic systems.

- **Analysing rework and the seven wastes**. Taiichi Ohno, one of the leading thinkers behind the Toyota Production System, describes Capacity as Work + Waste (Ohno, 1988, p. 21). Remove the waste, and you have the capacity to do more work. He goes on to identify seven forms of waste, which are often identified through process mapping and various forms of observation and work study. Ohno's seven wastes are:

  - **Overproduction**. In healthcare this could be overtreatment.
  - **Waiting**. Such as staff waiting for information, patients waiting for next steps etc.
  - **Transportation**. Avoidable movement of patients and equipment.
  - **Over-processing**. Ordering or requesting more of something due to lack of confidence in the system.
  - **Inventory**. See Chapter 5 for discussion on buffering the effects of variation with patients in beds (inventory).
  - **Movement**. Avoidable movement of staff.
  - **Rework**. The cost of poor quality and mistakes. Having to repeat process steps (re-ordering something, requesting information a second time).

Keeping Your Perspective When Exploring Detractors

While all of these activities are worthwhile, they are often applied without stepping back and viewing the bigger picture in terms of the scale of possible detractors. It is useful to consider detractors in terms of the timeframe they focus upon. For example the:

- year
- month
- week
- day.

All of the seven wastes, detailed in the previous paragraphs, are highly focused on the work done, the processes and the staff doing it – which is the level of the *day*. If focused on staff productivity (the level of the *day*), the very fact the staff member is at work masks much more sizable capacity detractors. Capacity losses and variation from planning decisions, policies and application of policy (or not) at the level of *year*, *month* and *week* are often far more sizable than the detractors at the level of the *day*. In a practical sense, a service could spend a huge amount of time chasing its tail trying to reduce detractors by a minute here or a minute there through using quality improvement tools, while through ineffective holiday, rota, sickness and training planning, a department could be, in our experience, up to 40% down on its entire capacity. At the level of the *week*, it is often legacies of part time working arrangements that mean certain days have more capacity than others – a pattern that often does not match the pattern of demand. While this is an emotive subject, and often one wrapped up in departmental and organisation politics, it is essential that capacity at the level of *year*, *month* and *week* is smoothed to reduce this highly impactful detraction from capacity – a level of detractor which hobbles departments at some periods during the year.

Reducing Failure Demand

Understanding and reducing Failure Demand is the often-forgotten tactic in reducing utilisation. Given traditionally far less attention, in its reduction there is dramatic potential impact on utilisation and thus delays. As shown in Figure 6.3, Failure Demand is the forgotten side of the utilisation equation, and it increases the demands services face.

$$Ut = \frac{\text{Value Demand} + \text{Failure Demand}}{\text{Base Capacity} - \text{Detractors}}$$

Figure 6.3   Strategies to reduce utilisation (Bicheno, 2012)

Failure Demand was brought into mainstream attention by leading improvement thinker John Seddon. He defines it as:

> The demand placed on the system, not as a result of delivering value to the "customer", but due to failings within the system. (Seddon, 2005)

In other words, in Failure Demand services are literally creating their own demand. This is not work generated by patient demand, but by their often counterproductive response to that demand. The list in Figure 6.4 details some examples.

- Having to request an additional appointment / see a patient again because a professional did not have the correct information.
- A patient escalating in their needs due to delays in their assessment / intervention / care plan.
- Spending time managing / resolving a patient complaint.
- Patients contacting a clinician / service as they are unclear on their next steps.
- Repeating assessments due to lack of information / confidence in the previous steps taken.
- Patients escalating in needs (perhaps presenting to other services) due to anxiety about next steps.
- Treating / helping a patient's initial presentation, rather than overall health / wellbeing.
- Overtreatment driven by medical / legal pressures.

(Downham, 2018)

Figure 6.4 Failure Demand examples

The scale of this, due to the size of most health and social care systems and providers, is considerable. Through GP-led demand studies of GP appointments, Develop Consulting, a primary care focused management consultancy, found that typically 10% of GP consults are directly a result of Failure Demand (Develop Consulting, 2022). This is an enormous figure given there were 158 million GP appointments in 2022 in the English NHS (NHS Digital, 2022).

The studies by Develop Consulting also highlighted that for 29% of patients who are frequent attenders, their current levels of complexity and need are a result of Failure Demand. Many of these patients will be those who are also attending more specialist services.

In secondary care, snapshot analysis in a large hospital setting has found failure demand to be just as present (Downham, 2023). For example, a clinician led snapshot audit[1] of ITU patients found 15% of patients to have an extended stay due to an avoidable clinical factor. An enormous figure when you consider the cost of ITU beds. In inpatient neuro / cardio rehab, a similar clinician led audit found that for 13% of patients their current complexity was a product of Failure Demand – defined as greater complexity caused by delays in the system. Moving to the specialty of psychiatry, a clinician led audit found 55% of patient cases being a product of Failure Demand – where again delays in the system have resulted in greater patient complexity that now requires a more complex and / or intensive intervention. A stark figure when you consider the pressure most mental health services are under.

It would be easy to say that these delays are just a product of lack of capacity, but this is not necessarily the case. Clinician led demand categorisation audit of key decision-making points in a large hospital setting, indicate other causes (Downham, 2023). For example, snapshot MDT meeting analysis suggests that in 25% of cases reviewed in neuro / cardiac rehabilitation MDT meetings, and 60% of cases in Psychiatric MDT meetings, a decision on next steps could not be made due to missing patient information and history, lack of confidence in previous assessment and / or expected diagnostics. Similar analysis of Radiology (supporting Emergency care in this instance), found that for 14% of cases referred the Radiologist was unable to make a judgement due to lack of information from the referrer. These examples illustrate not only a waste of a time (a capacity detractor) for expensive to convene groups of professionals, but more importantly potentially delaying the progress of the patient and increasing their complexity – creating Failure Demand.

The practical reality is that not only does this use precious resources, but it also means our efficiency-focused improvement efforts often concentrate on the wrong thing. We often rely on making capacity use more efficient (the capacity side of our utilisation equation) – or asking even more discretionary effort from our staff. But this opens up an important question – what if we are making the wrong work more efficient? What if we are asking our staff to use discretionary effort to meet demands that are avoidable in the first place?

Understanding Failure Demand is all about questioning the work in the first place.

Questioning the Work – Addressing Failure Demand

Failure Demand is not an individual issue. It is not about staff doing the wrong or right thing. It is about how the work has been designed, e.g. how healthcare systems, processes and organisations have been set up. The use of the word "design" is deliberate, because the way things are now is a result of a set of deliberate decisions. The good news is that, if leaders choose, a different set of design decisions can reduce the amount of Failure Demand created in the way services respond to patient need. In doing so delays and pressure can be reduced by reducing utilisation (without, incidentally, having to increase capacity).

Systems Deeply Shape the Way Work Is Done

From a sharp end service perspective, a legitimate question would be why do we tolerate this, in many cases, avoidable demand placed upon us? Why is it so normalised? Is it a public service attitude? That those inefficiencies are just accepted? Or could it be that individuals, especially those at the sharp end of delivery, have less influence over the causes than commonly thought?

There are deep-rooted reasons for our systems creating Failure Demand. These reasons are driven by the system conditions that effectively create the "rules of the game" when it comes to how individuals, teams and services respond to patient need. These are the official and unofficial forces that shape the work: policies, standards, guidelines, incentives, structures, information, targets, measurement, custom and practice, availability of equipment, resources, criteria, peer pressure and opinion – to name just a few. Leading leadership thinker Peter Senge describes how these system conditions influence behaviour – *individuals, however different, placed within the same structures (system conditions) will produce the same results* (adapted from Senge, 2006, p. 42). If leaders want individuals and teams to avoid Failure Demand, then they need to challenge these system conditions in which the work takes place – different design decisions have to be made.

Where staff members sit in an organisation or system determines their perspective, the influence the system has on them, and the influence they have on the system. Deming, in his core text *Out of Crisis* (Deming, 2000, p. 317), argues that leaders have a view of the system as explicit and definable. A leader may see the system as stakeholders, financial flows, regulation, employees, suppliers, patients, protocols, policy, other healthcare institutions, key performance indicators, key assets, facilities, information systems and so on. A leader may not have influence over all parts of this, but much of it they will.

For front line or more junior staff, the view of the system is quite different, and far less defined. To front line staff the system is, as Deming describes it, "everything but them". Their influence over it is smaller than that of a leader, although not negligible – they can still have influence on their own system of work in the choices they make. The lesson in this is that, if we want to reduce Failure Demand, we need to change the system conditions that create it – rather than think of it as predominantly an issue with individual employees. The people who hold "the keys" to these system conditions are leaders. It is leaders who hold much of the power in systems. John Seddon, in his text *Freedom from Command and Control* (Seddon, 2005), describes this relationship in his Thinking > System > Performance model. The performance (outcomes and approach to the work) is driven by the system (the system conditions – rules of the game), which in turn is shaped by the thinking – particularly of those with influence – leaders. Deming identified this thinking of leaders, their mental models, and gave it prominence in his writing. Most notably as the domain of Theory of Knowledge in his System of Profound Knowledge (Deming, 2018). The argument being leaders often have more power and agency than front line workers.

This arguably linear description of the cause and effect of leadership thinking and the shaping of front line system conditions, and thus the way work is done, provides a useful starting place for those wishing to fundamentally challenge and question the work done. But we must not forget that in practice, systems are far more complex and, frankly, messy. While front line staff have less influence, due to their reduced positional power, they can and do still act upon and shape their own system to a degree. They are less powerful but not powerless in questioning their own work. In the NHS there has been a growing interest in understanding systems in a more expansive, less linear, complexity-focused way with theories of Complex Adaptive Systems. In a useful evidence scan by the Health Foundation (The Health Foundation, 2010, p. 3), complex adaptive systems are defined as *an approach that challenges simple cause and effect assumptions and instead sees healthcare and other systems as dynamic. One where the interactions and relationships of different components simultaneously affect and are shaped by the system.* They argue that one of the roles of leadership is not only to shape the system, but also to learn to hold and work with the complexity of it. This counters the view that a leader's work is to control a system or elements of one. It suggests that many systems are so complex that attempts to control in a neat cause-and-effect manner are folly. That instead we as leaders should seek to enable the shaping and holding of complexity. You will see these themes in the coming chapters in our Principles to Avoid Failure Demand. where many of the principles enable better holding and working with complexity – that is, the complexity of the patient and their context, but also the complexity of our systems of healthcare delivery.

This discussion on systems is not proposing a binary choice between different systems theories, but rather identifying a progression. The contextualising and pragmatic introductions to systems and the power dynamic in systems from the likes of Deming and Seddon is hugely useful. They offer us a gateway into a progressive world of systems thinking – away from the atomising and individualising of the problems of healthcare. They help us begin to shape and question work in an actionable way. A way that is perhaps more tangible and actionable than complex adaptive systems theory, with the latter being sometimes seen as an "excuse not to strive to understand causes of organisational and social phenomenon" (The Health Foundation, 2010, p. 25). While we can recognise that some people are tempted to "admire the problem", we believe that with complexity theory you can better recognise and shape the causes of problems. Ultimately, this is about purpose and recognising the type of problem being faced. At this point it is useful to return to our three modes of organising we explored in Chapter 1. If we are seeking to move away from the *Mechanistic – Doing Things Better*[2] to modes of the *Participative – Doing Things Well* and the *Relational – Doing Better Things* (Anderson-Wallace et al., 2001) then systems thinking becomes important for the increasingly transformational change desired – with working with complexity being especially important in the latter.

Finally, it is important to recognise that just because something sounds mechanistic, it doesn't mean it is not useful in working systemically. These things can and should co-exist – they should not be seen as different tribes. Take, for example, the topic of variation explored in detail in Chapter 4. Despite its focus on the quantitative, on techniques and on rules, much of the thinking on variation helps us understand and act appropriately when faced with and working within complexity. For example, the notion of natural variation – as explored in the chapter, is complexity in action.

The Systemic Sources of Failure Demand in Healthcare

So what should happen in our systems to avoid Failure Demand? Failure Demand can manifest itself in many different ways (as illustrated previously in Figure 6.4), but the sources of these can be usefully themed into four distinct system conditions (as detailed in the four quadrants of Figure 6.5) (Downham, 2018). We propose these conditions need to change if we seek to reduce Failure Demand and lessen the pressure and delays on our systems of health and social care.

Fragmentation by Design	Defensive Pressures
• The fragmentation (dis-integration) of the work and services driven by industrial, economic, bureaucratic and professional ideologies	• Overtreatment driven by medical legal pressure, moral and ethical tensions, and fear of vilification • Short-term decision making and damaging subjective scrutiny driven by political ideology • Dehumanisation, objectification and mechanistic approaches driven by social system defences against anxiety (Menzies, 1960)
Specialist / Generalist Muddle	Misidentification of Needs
• Conducting generalist work in specialist settings • Generalists conducting specialist work • Turning skilled generalist work into specialist disciplines • Devaluation of the professional generalist	• Treating social as health • Treating health as social • Treating health presentations without addressing the underlying social causes • Designing health services with no social capability

Based on the original concept by Nick Downham (Downham, 2018)

Figure 6.5   Sources of Failure Demand in healthcare.

Fragmentation by Design

Esteemed healthcare thinker and physician Atul Gawande describes the challenge facing healthcare as one of complexity (Gawande, 2014). It is one of coordinating hugely complex responses to need, responses that consist of a vast number of contributions and connections. Every time there is a transition or handover between an individual, team, provider or even system there is a risk something falls between the cracks. These transitions are a de-coupling of care – de-coupling being a prime cause of Failure Demand (Seddon, 2005). With fragmented systems this de-coupling is on the increase. Some of this proliferation of the vast number of individuals, professions, specialists, teams and providers is driven by a genuine need for specialist input – especially where the boundaries of medical capability are being stretched. But some of this complexity is driven by other forces, such as economic, bureaucratic and professional ideologies that create further complexity and thus fragmentation.

Defensive Pressures

Defensive Pressures are a set of pressures that force clinicians, managers and staff to act upon a short-term view, or practise defensively, rather than take the long-term best interests of the service and patients. In many cases creating more work – Failure Demand. There are four broad groups of Defensive Pressures:

Medical/Legal

From a clinical perspective this can lead to overtreatment, excess diagnostics, depersonalisation and avoidable referring and deferring. This defensive practice is often driven by the perceived and/or actual medical/legal pressures, rather than the needs of the patient. In some settings, up to 93% of clinicians (Studdert et al., 2005) report practising defensively.

The Social Systems Defence against Anxiety

These Defensive Pressures are also driven by the social systems defence against anxiety among clinicians (Menzies, 1960). In the absence of effective mechanisms to support clinicians in the difficult and emotionally draining work of healthcare, they develop often extremely defensive strategies to protect themselves. These defences promote de-personalisation, avoidance of decisions, denial of feelings and even the breakdown of the patient/clinician relationship. All of these can potentially cause Failure Demand either in the setting in question, or elsewhere in systems.

Moral and Ethical Tensions

Clinicians are often torn between doing no harm to a patient and doing what is in their best interests. Complicating this balance is the increasing workload and medical/legal pressure clinicians face. Using the example of frailty, in some cases it is in the best interests and the wishes of the patient to remain at home, but they are admitted because of the potential risk of harm (perhaps there is a risk they may fall). This can in many cases lead to overtreatment, complications, and of course increased handovers – all sources of Failure Demand.

Political

Political ideologies come in all shapes and sizes, but there are dominant themes that lead to Failure Demand. Included in these is the push for short-term results. This pressure for results can often lead to changes to organisations that may be intended to improve a specific process or service but, in fact, just move the problem elsewhere. For example meeting the A&E four-hour wait, but just moving the pressure to elsewhere in the hospital or to community services. Another theme that emerges is the drive for personal accountability for what are systemic issues – or some would say "someone to blame". This forces leaders to look after their own interests, thus acting defensively, rather than seeing the whole and perhaps tackling the systemic causes of Failure Demand.

Specialist, Generalist and Citizen Muddle

Doing generalist work in specialist settings, doing specialist work in generalist settings, and doing both when in fact the citizen is better placed all cause Failure Demand. This plays out at many levels. For example:

- The interaction between a GP and a district hospital
- The relationship with the district hospital and the specialist/tertiary hospital
- The relationship between the consultant and nurse
- The relationship between a GP and the citizen and family

The scale of this is illustrated in a report by The Royal College of Paediatrics and Child Health that states that on average 33% of all PICU (specialist centre) bed days could have been cared for in local HDUs (Royal College of Paediatrics and Child Health, 2018). Continuing the theme, the high-profile NHS Getting It Right First Time reports for many of their comprehensive range of specialities studied found that inappropriate settings and referrals led to issues such as delays, avoidable admissions, re-admissions and the avoidable use of specialist input (see www.gettingitrightfirsttime.co.uk).

There are countless other examples. For example in community care there is the notion that all physical assessments must be done by a specialist or that social care assessments cannot be done by healthcare workers, or there are patients pressuring a GP, a highly skilled generalist clinician, to refer them to a specialist rather than managing their condition or presentation in the community – even if more appropriate.

Put simply, we frequently muddle generalist work (which still needs skill and a high level of expertise) with genuinely specialist work. It increases fragmentation, as it requires a larger number of different professionals and in the case of specialist centres, it drags patients unnecessarily away from their homes. It creates Failure Demand.

Misidentification of Needs

The social determinants of health dwarf the healthcare determinants of health – with social and environmental determinants having up to three times the impact on someone's health than healthcare services themselves (The King's Fund, 2012). Most clinicians accept this, that generally a health and social response is required to prevent and help someone with many of the chronic conditions common in our populations. Yet services are often set up with an overwhelming bias to a biomedical, or health, response. Of course, it does depend on the condition. For example, if a GP finds an indicator for cancer then it is appropriate and desirable to have a swift, reliable and effective response from the system. At least in the short term this will be health focused. But other conditions, such as type 2 diabetes, are much more dependent on a balanced mix of interventions – both health and social. It can often be social contextual pressure (life pressure) that undermines health advice and interventions (Downham, 2020).

This dominant health-focused design reduces options available to clinicians. Even if they identify a social need, they are often forced to misidentify it, in order to provide some form of support – for example prescribing anti-depressants for something that has social root causes. In other words, treating social as health. It forces clinicians to treat the presentation rather than the underlying cause. Hence clinicians watch, helplessly, as so many patients continue along a path of declining wellbeing while the clinician manages their individual presentations. Many of these individuals end up escalating in needs and complexity, requiring a very expensive intervention which could have been avoided if systems had the means of intervening differently – this is pure Failure Demand.

The chapters following will explore these four systemic sources in greater depth and propose some alternative system conditions and design principles, the antidotes to some of the Failure Demand we see in our services and systems.

Conclusions

In this and the previous chapter we started with the basic pressures that most healthcare systems face – that of quality, increasing delays and the call for greater productivity. In exploring a structured approach to solving these problems, through understanding the concept of utilisation and the influences upon it, we have explored powerful approaches in the struggle for greater productivity and flow. Namely the concepts of capacity detractors, and the far less well known concept of Failure Demand – both of which are driven by the important concept of variation. We then moved on to beginning our deep dive into the concept of Failure Demand – illustrating how our healthcare systems often literally make their own work.

The sources of this are systemic and often have strong socio-cultural considerations. We argue that this is not about individuals doing the wrong thing, but one of system conditions, the rules of the game, creating a system of work where individuals can do little different. Those who hold the greater share of the influence on these system conditions are leaders. It is the ideologies and beliefs of leaders, about how things should be, that create many of these conditions. This is aptly summarised in an old Toyota saying "that the shop floor is a reflection of management" (Bicheno, 2012, p. 101).

It is easy to see what is being explored in this Chapter, and the one before it, as a set of hard truths or answers, as the language used, often by the original authors of the concepts, is very direct and the linear nature very compelling. While these concepts are very useful in beginning to piece together and make sense of complex interconnected systems and their actions, it is important to note that that same complexity itself requires nuanced consideration. For example it would be an error to consider the "system" as something separate to oneself when working within a complex system such as healthcare services. Professionals, staff and leaders are all influenced by the system of work they are within, and influence it in the same breath – especially as they become more influential. This means the answers are never neat, and staff always have some influence and choice. So perhaps the best way to think about these conceptual models, often from authors whose thinking first originated from more mechanistic backgrounds, is as useful prompts rather than hard and fast rules. These concrete sounding models and rules provide a useful set of variables or prompts to help recognise things the system of healthcare delivery should consider when putting together a hypothesis for change. Prompts that will leave those who use them in a far better position than if not used at all. They are prompts that require contextualisation nevertheless, and being flexible and adaptive in learning and responding to the likely outcomes in their use is important.

To conclude, and to position the remaining chapters, we have introduced four Systemic Sources of Failure Demand. These four interconnected themes, we argue, to a great extent account for the Failure Demand in our healthcare systems. If services want to address the rising demands and pressures of productivity, without the only option being investing in more capacity, then services and systems need to consider and begin to address these sources of avoidable demands. The four Systemic Sources of Failure Demand introduced – Fragmentation by Design; Defensive Pressures; The Generalist, Specialist and Citizen Muddle; and Misidentification of Need – provide a powerful lens to do so, reminding services that not all of the demands faced, and the resulting work done, is from the patient's original needs. The current NHS system, and many like it, makes meeting need and thus reducing demand harder, slower and more costly than it needs to be.

The first step in all of this is to have the humility, direction and headspace to *challenge the existing assumptions of healthcare delivery, to question the work,* in the first place.

Acknowledgements

We would like to thank Jo Gibson, Brendan O'Donovan and John Seddon for sharing their expertise, in their writing and in person, in the concept of Failure Demand. We would also like to thank Dr Iolanthe Fowler, Dr Ollie Hart, Chris Easton, Simon Bricknell, Max Pardo-Roques, Steve Boam and Tony Hufflet for their contribution to shaping our thinking on the implications and form of Failure Demand in healthcare.

Notes

1 A snapshot analysis involves senior clinicians using a demand categorisation audit tool to create a single point in time (snapshot) picture of all of the cases in a care setting.
2 The domain of Quality Control as described by Juran (1989).

References

Anderson-Wallace, M., Blantern, C. and Boydell, T. 2001. Advances in cross-boundary practice: Inter-logics as a method. *Career Development International*, 6(7): 414–420.

Berwick, D. 2008. A transatlantic review of the NHS at 60. *BMJ*, 337: 212. www.bmj.com/bmj/section-pdf/186530?path=/bmj/337/7663/Analysis.full.pdf

Bicheno, J. 2012. *The Service Systems Toolbox*. Picsie Books.

Deming, W.E. 2000. *Out of Crisis*. MIT Press.

Deming, W.E. 2018. *The New Economics* (3rd edn). The MIT Press.

Develop Consulting. 2022. *General Practice Opportunity Search*. Develop Consulting Ltd.

Downham, N. 2018. *Sources of Failure Demand in Healthcare*. www.cressbrookltd.co.uk/sources-of-failure-demand-in-healthcare/

Downham, N. 2020. *The Reality of Patient Context in General Practice*. www.cressbrookltd.co.uk/the-reality-of-social-context-gp/

Downham, N. 2023. Assessment of Failure Demand in a Large Hospital Setting. June 2023. Unpublished.

Gawande, A. 2014. *BBC Radio 4 – The Reith Lectures*. www.bbc.co.uk/programmes/b04sv1s5

Gilbreth, F.B. and Gilbreth, L.M. 1910–1919. *Motion Study and Time Study Instruments of Precision*. Available in the Royal College of Surgeons of England / Wellcome Collection. https://wellcomecollection.org/works/cngbu9a4

Hirano, H. 1995. *5 Pillars of the Visual Workplace*. Productivity Press.

Hopp, W. and Spearman, M. 2000. *Factory Physics* (2nd edn). McGraw-Hill.

Juran, J.M. 1989. *Juran on Leadership for Quality – An Executive Handbook*. Free Press.

Menzies, I.E.P. 1960. A case-study in the functioning of social systems as a defence against anxiety: A report on a study of the nursing service of a general hospital. *Tavistock Institute for Human Relations*, 13(2): 95–121.

NHS Digital. 2022. *Appointments in General Practice, December 2022*. https://digital.nhs.uk/data-and-information/publications/statistical/appointments-in-general-practice/december-2022

NHS Institute for Innovation and Improvement. 2008. *Releasing Time to Care: The Productive Ward – Toolkit*. NHS Institute for Innovation and Improvement.

Ohno, T. 1988. *Toyota Production System – Beyond Large-Scale Production*. Taylor and Francis.

Royal College of Paediatrics and Child Health. 2018. *High Dependency Care for Children – Time to Move On*. www.rcpch.ac.uk/sites/default/files/2018-07/high_dependency_care_for_children_-_time_to_move_on.pdf

Seddon, J. 2005. *Freedom from Command and Control* (2nd edn). Vanguard Education Ltd.

Senge, P. 2006. *The Fifth Discipline – The Art and Practice of the Learning Organisation* (2nd edn). Random House Business Books.

Shingo, S. 1985. *A Revolution in Manufacturing, the SMED System*. Productivity Press.

Shingo, S. 1987. *Key Strategies for Plant Improvement* (English translation edn by Andrew P. Dillon). Productivity Press.

Studdert D.M., Mello, M.M., Sage, W.M., DesRoches, C.M., Peugh, J., Zapert, K. and Brennan, T.A. 2005. Defensive medicine among high-risk specialist physicians in a volatile malpractice environment. *JAMA*, 293(21): 2609–2617.

The Health Foundation, 2010. *Evidence Scan: Complex Adaptive Systems*. The Health Foundation.

The King's Fund. n.d. *How Much Has Been Spent on the NHS since 2005?* www.kingsfund.org.uk/projects/general-election-2010/money-spent-nhs

The King's Fund. 2012. *Broader Determinants of Health: Future Trends*. www.kingsfund.org.uk/projects/time-think-differently/trends-broader-determinants-health

Taylor, F.W. 2005. *The Principles of Scientific Management*. 1st World Library.

Wennberg, J. 2002. Unwarranted variations in healthcare delivery: Implications for academic medical centres. *BMJ*, 325: 961–964.

7

Principles to Avoid Failure Demand

Framing

In Chapter 6 we introduced four Sources of Failure Demand in Healthcare. These were:

- Fragmentation by Design
- Defensive Pressures
- The Specialist, Generalist and Citizen Muddle
- Misidentification of Needs

Our argument is that these sources of Failure Demand need to be recognised and acted upon to enhance quality and thus improve efficiency into our systems of work. These are broad categories that we have identified as significant stumbling blocks that appear to hold back many healthcare systems in their efforts to respond to growing demand and changing patterns of disease and need.

In Figure 7.1, we present a model featuring four domains, and principles within them, which based on our practical experience and empirical research are important to consider in response to the sources of Failure Demand identified in the previous chapter.

Defragmenting to Integrate	Supporting Human Systems at Work:
• Simplify (defragment) system design rather than overlay extra communication. • Highly skilled generalist teams in primary care, designed to avoid having to defer and refer. Able to do '80% of everything' • Self-directed. • Point costing replaced by population and end to end costing. • Proactive in nature. • The community is part of the team. • Assessments to increase knowledge rather than gate keep. • Reduced proliferation of new roles, specialisms and professionals.	Recognize the effect of the strange moral and psychological world of healthcare: • Appreciate social systems defences against anxiety. • Promote the conditions for interpersonal risk and organisational health. • Institutional reflective practice and restorative approaches.
Avoiding the Specialist, Generalist and Citizen Muddle:	Understanding Need
• Generalists valued as much as specialists. • Specialists support (consult in) to generalists (or whoever holds the relationship with the patient) wherever appropriate. • Seek to avoid referring and deferring – maximum subsidiarity • The professions promote broadening of responsibilities towards 'doing what matters' • Frameworks and governance support professionals to do a wider span of activities. • Mechanisms in place to keep work in more general / non specialist settings wherever possible.	• Designing the work to do 'what matters' rather than 'what fits'. • Harnessing the flexibility and creativity in person-centred approaches. • Understanding the difference between relational and linear work. • Realize the power of social context.

Based on the original concept by Nick Downham (Downham, 2018)

Figure 7.1   Principles to avoid Failure Demand in Healthcare
Anderson-Wallace and Downham 2023

In the chapters that follow, we will be exploring these domains and the issues that require consideration, including reviewing and where necessary reframing some of the ideological positions and belief systems that shape them. Within this we draw on the available evidence and illustrate with practical examples.

The Role of the Domains and Principles Within Them

We propose that these domains, and principles within them, are used to challenge dominant assumptions of healthcare delivery – to help question the work. That they are used to generate focus and to promote curiosity, inquiry and reflection.

They can be used to organise and structure design and review activities, but also as reference points for more continuous and organic reflection. Critically, we do not present them as a complete answer. They are positioned as a useful heuristic – to guide discussion; to promote learning and discovery; and to help challenge traditional thinking – between people involved and affected by the work.

Over many years there has been a strong focus on the need for new models of care, but it is very telling that most of the time these new models look remarkably like the old ones. Our invitation is to use these domains to avoid that trap. We recognise that these domains will be improved upon, refined and reframed, but in their current form we think they provide busy people some structure and knowledge to base their questioning of work upon.

8

Defragmenting to Integrate

In Chapter 7 we proposed a framework featuring four domains of Principles to Avoid Failure Demand. The four domains within the framework were:

- Defragmenting to Integrate
- Avoiding the Specialist, Generalist and Citizen Muddle
- Supporting Human Systems at Work
- Understanding Need

This chapter focuses on the first of these domains, as illustrated in Figure 8.1, on the principles of simplified and proactive models of care that integrate and overcome the fragmentation (dis-integration) of the work and services.

- Simplify (defragment) system design rather than overlay extra communication
- Highly skilled generalist teams in primary care, designed to avoid having to defer and refer. Able to do '80% of everything'
- Self-directed
- Point costing replaced by population and end-to-end costing
- Proactive in nature
- The community is part of the team
- Assessments to increase knowledge rather than gate keep
- Reduced proliferation of new roles, specialisms and professionals

---

Figure 8.1 Defragmenting to Integrate

Fragmentation is everywhere in our systems of healthcare. In all but the simplest of interventions, care often involves many professionals, many professions, many departments, several providers and sometimes even different sectors – such as health, social and the charity/voluntary sector. A frail elderly person may see, in one month, a number of different GPs, several different community nurses, a care assessor, multiple carers, an occupation therapist, equipment providers and dieticians. If they have a short inpatient stay in that period, countless ward staff, geriatricians, discharge coordinators and care package assessors can be added to the count. The list could go on and is at minimum very confusing for the individual. All of this has the very real potential to fragment care. This fragmentation can cause confusion, repetition, delay, gaps in service delivery and can even result in people getting lost in systems of care (Monitor, 2015).

As we discussed in Chapter 6, de-coupling (Seddon, 2005) of the delivery of care, characterised by handovers and transitions, are a prime source of Failure Demand. Fragmentation of care delivery being a big driver of the volume of handovers and transitions in many patients' care. The consequences of this fragmentation of care can be seen in detail in Figure 8.2.

- **Dilution of responsibility.** The more professionals that are involved in something, the less clear the responsibility. When everyone is responsible – the chances are no one is.
- **Transitions and handovers.** Each time information, responsibility and patients transition between individuals, systems, teams and providers there is a risk that what is important falls between the cracks. This creates Failure Demand.
- **Sub optimisation.** Typically, each team, department and service has its own key performance indicators, budgets and incentives. These drive the individual parts to optimise themselves – often to the detriment of other parts of the system and thus the system as a whole. This is one of the main reasons hospital costs overall continue to rise, despite relentless cost improvement programmes and measures.
- **Increased variability.** Each moving part will have its own inherent variability – potentially causing the requirement to buffer with either extended timelines, capacity or work in process (typically patients in beds waiting).
- **Increased complexity.** This increases the chances of safety events and also makes the task of coordination more difficult. Hugely expensive IT systems, and single points of access are often the response to the increased communications challenge that surfaces with more complex systems.

Figure 8.2   Consequences of fragmentation

Responding to Fragmentation

Of course, the obvious response to fragmentation is integration. True integration means the unity of effort (Lawrence & Lorsch, 1967) in a system. The cause of many of the barriers to this unity of effort is the, arguably deliberate, fragmentation of systems of health and care.

Integration is a hot topic in most health systems and has been for decades. The fact that it has been for decades tells us something – that integration is exceedingly difficult, and in many cases integration efforts have not delivered the desired improvements. In fact, often things have got worse.

The following telling letter to the editor in the *BMJ*, in response to the introduction of divisional structures into hospitals in the English NHS, following the Joint Working Party on the Organisation of Medical Work in Hospitals in 1972 (also known as the Cogwheel report), could have been written just yesterday when considering the challenges still faced by many modern health systems. Integration is still a long way from being achieved.

Integrated hospital services

Sir – Four years after the publication of the "Cogwheel" report progress towards implementation has been patchy and mainly uninspired. Perhaps because the concept is wrong. One of the major problems facing medicine throughout the so-called developed world is increasing specialisation and fragmentation. Talk of improving communications and better liaison between different divisions and sub-divisions is little more than talk. The family doctor is rarely in close touch with the hospital specialists, who, in turn, are often isolated from each other. In spite of limited resources in manpower, money and buildings and equipment, services are often duplicated, and individual skills misused or neglected. (BMJ, 1972)

Perhaps the reason for this historic difficulty is not lack of effort, but because we don't tackle the core issues. We instead try to cope with the symptoms caused by lack of integration, rather than seek to understand and begin to address the reasons why they might be so fragmented in the first place.

When it comes to integration efforts, we often see:

- Co-location
- Merging or taking over organisations (consolidation). Vertical or horizontal integration
- Introduction of system overview systems (control systems)
- Communication systems (IT led)
- Communication and planning through MDT-style forums – towards integrated care
- Clinical system integration
- Communication and referral rationalisation such as a single point of access
- Financial (pooled budgets)

- Pathway management
- Skill mix changes
- Joint assessments and more holistic assessments

It could be argued that many of these initiatives are sticking plasters to a response to need which is too complicated, and has too many moving parts to manage – that is fragmented.

Take the example of single point of access (SPA) from the list. SPA systems are often overlaid onto complex and fragmented care systems in order to improve communication and cut down on confusion across the large number of parties involved. Picking up on the previous example of a frail person's care, a single telephone number, often handled by a call centre or hub with clinical support, coordinates requests for help from patients and professionals with the aim of connecting the right professionals to the patient. The aim of this process is to reduce things like avoidable admissions.

Simplified and Proactive

This all seems entirely logical when considering the often-cited aim of improving communication – but what if the response to need did not involve so many parties? Would communication be easier and more reliable if there were fewer moving parts in the first place? This illustrates the core principle of designing a response to need with the fewest parties, providers and individuals involved as possible – whilst still being effective. Fewer moving parts means fewer handovers and transitions. Fewer transitions reduces the risk of Failure Demand (Seddon, 2005).

To reduce the number of parties involved in an effective response to need, we need to question the perspective they view the work from. Traditionally we seek to fit the patient into existing structures. Yet to simplify but maintain or improve the effectiveness of response while doing so, there is more value in organising around the patient. An important step in doing so is to consider why we are structured the way we are, that is with a huge number of parties involved in meeting need.

To be clear at this stage, it is not an argument that applies to every patient, especially those with high clinical complexity; their need is such that the only way to respond effectively is by involving another party – typically a specialist. This could be a referral to a specialist, or a request for a specialist to attend the patient, the specialist having the required knowledge, capability and mandate, in a certain aspect of the patient's need.

The key consideration is what is driving this positioning of mandate, knowledge and capability? Certainly, much of it is down to quality and effectiveness, but as we will explore, there are other "forces" at play that drive this positioning, mandate and thus requirement for a transition or handover.

The forces that drive this can be thought of as the ideologies, or beliefs. As W. Edwards Deming suggests in his Theory of Profound Knowledge (Deming, 2018) it is often the Theory of Knowledge (ideology) of leaders that governs how services are designed. These ideologies are often unspoken and unrecognised as they are so normalised. We often just assume that this is how the organisational world works. We get taught them in many university courses and business schools, and implicitly in most medical training.

Ideologies That Fragment

For the purposes of this discussion we have grouped the ideologies that can often have the effect of proliferating division and specialisation, beyond the needs of clinical effectiveness and quality and thus fragmenting into three themes:

- Economic
- Bureaucratic
- Professional(ism)

The influence of economic thinking has been profound in health services. It is in the DNA of most healthcare systems. Of particular emphasis is the concentration on reducing labour costs, which is unsurprising given the proportion of service budgets that typically account for staff costs. In the English NHS in 2019/2020, this was £56.1 billion (King's Fund, 2022). A key strategy for reducing labour costs, and of relevance here, is the division of labour. This is the process of dividing work and job roles into smaller parts that can be simplified, specified and controlled. It means that an otherwise complex role can be split up into parts so someone lower skilled can do a piece of the work and/or can specialise in a certain type of work. This has been demonstrated, especially in the industrial context, to have a profound effect on reducing the labour costs overall. The lineage of this thinking goes back to the works of the hugely influential, and to the same extent polarising, Scottish economist and philosopher Adam Smith in the 18th century (Smith, 1776). Smith's ideas are widely credited as the foundations for modern economics and industrial thinking – the impact of which can be felt in everyone's lives.

Division of labour can be seen everywhere in health and social care. From the proliferation of different nursing roles on a ward, to the outsourcing of some roles and tasks, to the splitting up of care into tasks involving multiple professions and professionals. For example, at any one time on a ward there could be a ward sister, staff nurses, nursing assistants, ward clerks, junior doctors, a senior staff nurse, a senior nursing assistant, domestics (often outsourced), volunteers, housekeepers, a matron and discharge coordinators. All of these professionals are specialists in that they have their own area of focus – mandate, knowledge and capability. So far so good if this is driven by genuine quality and effectiveness, but if this is driven by economic division of labour, then potentially risks emerge – risks such as dilution of responsibility, task focus and losing sight of the ward as a system. From a cost perspective, the point cost (sometimes called the touch point cost) might be lower as roles are divided up and focused on more specific tasks. The acid test is whether the end-to-end cost – the cost over the complete episode of care, including primary care elements, also reduces. For this to reduce, the episode of care must be effective over time. If the overall episode is not effective, then while the point costs (the tasks) might be lower, the overall result of the entire episode might be higher. It is entirely possible for the point costs to go down, but overall costs (end to end) to creep up.

Much of this division of labour is driven by the notion of economies of scale. The summary argument being that if we concentrate on fewer things and do more of them it will be cheaper. Concentrating labour, through division of roles, on more prescribed and specified tasks also allows for the greater control of the tasks. It allows for a more scientific or perhaps industrial approach to tasks – allowing them to be documented and studied with the view to making them more efficient. It also allows them to be audited, potentially helping to increase reliability, provide a mechanism for control and potentially reduce variability (see Chapter 4) – something which many systems place great value on. Finally, the division and specifying of tasks allows lower skilled workers to undertake them, as the task can be described and trained – it even potentially allows for outsourcing of tasks. To enable all of this, work needs to be labelled. These labelled needs (Davis, 2016) can then be allocated to staff to be met in the specified way. This may work smoothly if needs and labels match, but is extremely problematic if they don't. Just because the need does not match does not mean there is no need – so either the person gets turned away, potentially creating further interactions and Failure Demand later down the line, or the clinician must distort the picture to somehow fit the need into the label – compromising the subsequent effectiveness of the response.[1]

The idea of enabling the control of the work through division of labour is central to the second ideological theme – that of bureaucratic design. This is not a simplistic view of bureaucracy, such as excess paperwork, but rather a set of intricate and deliberate principles on which many institutions and systems are designed. Many of these principles overlap with the ideas from economic thinking explored previously. The codification of bureaucratic design that we recognise in many of our structures today, in its purest form, comes in no small part from the thinking of the economist and sociologist Max Weber. In his work *Economy and Society* (Weber, 2013), first published posthumously in 1922, he detailed many of the principles of modern bureaucracy that have shaped the civil service, large business and healthcare systems globally. When we think of a traditional organisational form, what we visualise are bureaucratic design principles in action. So engrained are these principles, they are often not discussed or even brought to the surface. Even as they have begun to be questioned, as systems and services struggle with the challenges of complexity, the original promise of such a bureaucratic system as stated by Weber – that of precision, speed, unambiguity, knowledge of the files (the internal process), continuity, discretion, unity, strict subordination, reduction of friction and of material and personal costs (Weber, 2013, p. 973) – remain hugely attractive to leaders, and so the principles remain visible in many organisations (Kennedy, 2007).

Weber's characteristics of modern bureaucracy are:

- Functional specialisation and division of labour: Described by Weber as the principle of jurisdictional areas, officials (workers) concentrate tightly on their area of specialisation and remit - and theirs only. They don't get involved in the work of others. This limits spans of influence and control. Crucially this involves determining the mandate of different professionals - determining the work they can and cannot do.
- Clear hierarchy: Ensuring a clearly defined system of subordination and superordination. With clear supervision of lower offices (roles) by higher ones. Weber stresses that monocratic hierarchy is important - where one person is clearly responsible for a specific task.
- Written documents (the files): To remove ambiguity, increase accountability and reliance on individuals and the overall process, all tasks within and all steps taken are documented.
- Specialisation: The offices (functions/departments) that make up the organisation are to become highly specialised through training. These functions can sometimes be highly recognisable across different institutional bureaucracies even in different sectors. Functions such as finance, office of the executive, human resources etc.
- General rules: Management of offices (functions) follow rules that are stable, exhaustive and can be taught and learned. These are the norms, processes and decision-making processes that drive the bureaucracy.
- Removing emotion: The discharge of the "business" of the bureaucracy without regard for persons. For example, the removal of privilege normally afforded by status. This is done in the most part through the creation of calculable rules (this could be criteria in many healthcare settings) that are discharged in a de-humanised manner - that is eliminating love, hatred, personal and irrational elements from the decision.

(Adapted from Weber, 2013, pp. 956-975)

To a greater or lesser extent, the shadows of Weber's thinking can be seen across our healthcare institutions. The tight focus of different professionals, the prescribed processes, the role of professional management as a discipline itself, the mechanisation of care, the governance processes and the decision-making processes are all commonly found. There is no argument that this brings stability and mechanisms to govern. It allows for control – something required in large institutions. It also brings, along with Adam Smith's thinking, the promise of more efficiency – by being able to concentrate resources on highly specified work and processes.

Despite this it is important to reflect upon this drive for division of labour, high levels of accountability and specification – with how this has panned out, in reality, in our complex systems of healthcare. Despite the advantages as proposed by Smith, Weber and other proponents of these principles, it has to be noticed that in complex systems of healthcare there is a curious but profoundly damaging paradox; that while massive levels of task specification, accountability and control have been created, in many systems there has been a loss of control, accountability and visibility of the whole. In many cases care has been atomised to the point where we are blind to the whole. Using the example of care of those who are frail, despite the large numbers of professionals involved, it is extremely hard to determine who is responsible. Divided responsibility can often lead to no responsibility (Deming, 2000, p. 30) and even when someone is identified as responsible, they often have little practical authority or agency to act on the activities of others involved in other care tasks. The efficient, specified and governed touch points or tasks often don't add up to an effective whole.

There is a strong argument that these methods have helped drive efficiency, reliability and accessibility in industrial and many public services. They have been an important part in the improvements in our living standards and healthcare outcomes. But as healthcare gets more complex, driven by changing patterns of ill health, ageing populations and advances in medical knowledge, the cracks are emerging and the "promise" of continued efficiency is more and more elusive. To achieve a high level of quality and thus efficiency it is not a case of a binary choice of design principles – economic/bureaucratic ideologies or not – but rather it is an exercise in balance and understanding of the true nature of the work, achieved by questioning the work done. These ideas that currently dominate nearly all types of healthcare organisation are perhaps more effective for certain types of work than others – with certain types of work they are counterproductive. A useful simple starting typology would be to distinguish the work of healthcare into two categories. That of Linear and Relational.

- **Linear work** is largely process driven and bio-medical, such as a test in secondary care, drug, seeing a clinical specialist, medical assessment or medical procedure (Downham, 2020). These can be highly technical in nature but success is generally reliant on technical process steps coming together with timeliness and high reliability, applying known knowledge and process well.
- **Relational work** may include the biomedical, but it is largely reliant on factors outside the bio-medical, such as the person's network, environment and social circumstance (Downham, 2020).

The use of economic and bureaucratic ideas is much better suited to work that is Linear in nature – work that is much more highly defined and boundaried. Where we know what is required, and we need to do it reliably and well. Where the work contains high proportions of the Relational,[2] these ideas come unstuck when applied too purely. The challenge is that the same episode of care may transition between highly linear and relational periods of work – where different organising approaches are required.

The last ideological theme to overlay on this picture of increasing fragmentation is that of professionalism. In this case referring to the role of and ideas behind the professions. The professions are as old as the idea of organised healthcare itself and they play important roles in our systems of care. They define and uphold minimum standards, define education, protect integrity and confidence in the profession, share best practice and work to maintain the status and renumeration of their members. Over time the number of professions has grown as the number of specialisms has grown. In the English NHS there are in excess of 270 different professions (NHS Health Careers, n.d.), many of which have professional bodies. Much of this is a response to the rapidly increasing volume of medical knowledge. In 2020 the doubling time of medical knowledge was forecast to be 73 days – such is the rapid advancement of knowledge (Dansen, 2011). Without effective decision support tools for clinicians, the volume of knowledge drives the need to specialise. Another factor driving the proliferation of professions is the perceived status of a specialist. The public feel more reassured in the hands of a perceived specialist. So different specialists seek to be recognised as their own profession, complete with professional body.

While much of this direction of travel towards specialism by the professions can be of great value, the impact on fragmentation should not be ignored. The increasing number of specialisms, driven often by professional ideologies, produces fragmentation and barriers to integration. It does so for two reasons. The first has the same effect as division of labour. The unintended consequence of the professions seeking to protect and determine the boundaries of their roles to protect their members is the creation of boundaries between professions. For a large part, these are important as it helps maintain quality – but this can also increase the number of transitions involved in patient care. The second reason is the professions can be a limiting factor in efforts to change models of care to suit changes in patterns of disease and demand. In working to protect their members from increasing demands or erosion of status, they potentially limit innovation. Especially when the greatest challenge we face is one of complexity and interconnectivity (Gawande, 2014), one of integration of work – something that if done effectively will always involve challenging existing role boundaries.

Integration – Defragmenting the Work

As discussed, these three ideological themes, or dominant ideas, can create forces that fragment work through the division of labour, the creation of firm boundaries, the limiting of mandate and the establishment of hard hierarchy. This deliberate fragmentation is not done in the belief that it will make things worse. It is done in the, often unwavering, belief that this is how things should be.

Simplified and Proactive

For true integration, that is a system with unity of purpose (Lawrence & Lorsch, 1967), we need to question these long-held assumptions on how organisations "should be". Instead of just focusing on "joining up", we argue true integration should also adopt the principle of seeking the simplest response to need first. This means the fewest number of professionals and thus handovers possible, rather than looking for mechanisms to coordinate a potentially already over-complicated response. This seeking of simplicity should not be confused with ignoring the complexity of care, but rather it is this simplicity, using highly empowered, skilled and widely mandated teams, that enables the holding of complexity. A key enabler to this is the notion of the highly skilled generalist – which challenges existing role and professional boundaries, where traditionally we fit need (which is often misidentified – see Chapter 11) by labelling it into the existing professional structures. With the notion of the highly skilled generalist we start with need first, and then determine the competencies required. Working to create a skill mix that fits the majority of the need.

80% of Everything and the Community as Part of the Team

The core principle of the work of Vifredo Pareto, creator of the Pareto principle – otherwise known as the 80/20 rule, a set of principles and techniques that was developed into the form widely recognised today by Joseph Juran (1989; Juran – Attain Partners, 2019) – provides a useful goal when considering skill mix. That is to work towards creating a role, or the simplest possible small team that can do 80% of everything – leaving only 20% to other specialists. Picking up on the example of care of someone who is frail and housebound, during a design exercise we were involved in with an urban health system, it was possible to list all the competencies required to look after someone holistically so that one role could do 80% of everything – from a health and social perspective. These competencies included care activities, wound care, limited prescribing, being a trusted assessor, activities of daily living, food prep, nursing tasks, nutrition, feeding and mobility. This would currently be the responsibility of tens of different professionals but it was not a big leap to design one role, with the right access to guidance if required, that was capable of fulfilling 80% of everything – reducing the need for handovers and the risk of Failure Demand. The interesting thing was the nearest role that matched these competencies was a traditionally structured district nursing role once seen in large numbers in the NHS – before the three dominant ideologies took hold to the extent seen today.

In starting to think about this, it is important to consider the family unit and the community as central to good outcomes, and thus part of the team, with most conditions. This is especially important if we want a more proactive model of care. For example, in the celebrated Buurtzorg model of integrated nursing led home care, discussed in more detail later in this chapter, the first tier of support is the family and community. The nursing teams actively engage and support communities to support those who need it wherever possible, before considering providing that support themselves (Jansen, 2023).

Many of these simpler, relational in focus and defragmented ways of working already exist in some health systems. In the much-celebrated Brazilian Family Health System community healthcare workers, supported by a GP and nurse, who consults in to support them, have a portfolio of responsibilities and matching competencies that enable them to look after the majority of a family's health and social needs (Commonwealth Fund, 2016). In the English NHS this portfolio would typically involve ten or more different professions and even more individual professionals. The result is less fragmentation and less reliance on hospitals than other healthcare systems (Britnell, 2015). To achieve 80% of everything, for a simpler response to need, for relational work that requires it, we need to relax the hold of the dominant, common ideas that reinforce the current system. In targeted parts of our systems there is a need to relax the division of labour and create highly skilled generalist professionals and support them with on-hand specialist advice when required – rather than having to refer the patient to get this advice. The much-heralded Intermountain primary care mental health pathway improvements (Intermountain Healthcare, 2016) has resulted in successes such as 7% reduced primary care encounters and 10.6% reduction in hospital admissions for patients with mental health problems. Improvements in decision support systems and more timely support for professionals (Healthcare, 2018) has meant primary care professionals can hold more complex patients without the need to refer to specialists – avoiding transitions.

This means different things in different settings such as primary or secondary care. The term generalist does not mean lesser skilled – in fact it means a wider portfolio of skills – something to be highly valued. It means a set of competencies that fall outside of one existing profession or role. This challenges us to think innovatively about systems of professional accountability and governance – existing mechanisms that are set up for models of care that increasingly no longer suit the patterns of disease and demands faced. Of course, challenging existing role definitions is not just a managerial task – it is a challenge for the professions themselves. "Integration will not deliver benefits if clinicians do not change the way they work"

(Ham & Curry, 2011, p. 2). There is growing public opinion that some of the reason the English NHS is so resistant to reform is the pyramid of professional protectionism that exists (Jenkins, 2022).

Challenging Assessments

Assessments are the bread and butter of health and social care systems. They occur at intervals in the care cycle and during transitions between professionals, teams and services. They are used to create knowledge – such as to determine status and eligibility. As experienced by anyone working within these settings, or a patient subject to them, assessments can also slow down care and fragment. They generally require a particular professional to do them and may also introduce a process of sign-off due to structures of hierarchy – such as for a care package. When trying to improve integration an important step is to question the value of the assessment – why is there one? And if required, does it need a new (to the patient's care) professional to do it? Where assessments cause problems for integration is when they are used to gatekeep or when they are undertaken because a professional does not have trust in the previous assessment, even if the timeframe and the previous professional's competency is valid. This is driven in part by Defensive Pressures (see Chapter 10). Creating a system where professionals can trust each other enough to avoid a proportion of repeated assessments can simplify things and thus improve integration.

Gatekeeping is used to check if a patient meets criteria – often even when another professional has made that determination in the referral. This gatekeeping could be to protect capacity, although this invariably just causes patients with more developed symptoms to present later (Failure Demand), due to the need to authorise a transition – which is often the case if funding is involved. These assessments and subsequent sign-off steps are a form of inspection in hierarchies, where decision making is separated from the work, and lower levels are subordinate to higher levels. It is questionable whether multiple sign-offs add any value or rigor – as all that happens with multiple signatories is each defaults to the previous (Deming, 2000, p. 30).

Self-Directed

The final principles in this simplified and proactive approach to integration are focused on relaxing the tight grasp on control and remit. As found to be a key pillar in the incredibly successful Buurtzorg model of homecare, self-directed teams have been shown to produce huge quality and cost benefits. Counter intuitively, the cost savings come not solely from the front line touch point (the hourly cost), but rather in the resulting reduction in back office costs due to creating self-directed teams with high levels of autonomy. Buurtzorg's 8000+ nurses require just 50 back office staff and managers (Jansen, 2019) (Britnell, 2015, p. 180). This has been achieved by vastly reducing the levels of subordination and resulting permission processes, reversing division of labour (increasing scope) and increasing the spans of control of front line teams. This proves that with less hierarchical control, costs don't have to run away – in fact they can reduce.

More agency and autonomy can also help other pressures that our systems face. Of particular challenge to the English NHS, staff retention, or lack thereof, is causing serious pressure and threatening continuity of services. It is also an avoidable waste of money with the training cost of a doctor being £230,000 (HM Government, 2017). In addition to pay and pension issues, doctors cite loss of respect, lack of value and fragmented teamwork as reasons for leaving or considering leaving (BMJ, 2020). Allowing clinicians to have more autonomy is perhaps part of the answer to reducing the trend of clinicians leaving.

Conclusions

Finding the right balance between control and autonomy is not something that only healthcare services wrestle with. Peter Wickens, former HR director of the consistently successful Nissan UK, describes the intricate balance between governance (*control*) and *engagement* (commitment of the people) in his book *The Ascendant Organisation* (Wickens, 1998). Too much *control* and you alienate, too little and you have anarchy. Get the balance right, and organisations ascend. For the English NHS this balance is rarely if ever found. The pendulum swings harshly between the two ends of the spectrum, often driven by political response to crisis or scandal rather than in any planned way. Over the past decade, it has been *control* that has been the emphasis – suggesting the three ideological themes discussed in this chapter are getting more dominant.

What we have proposed in this chapter is that the notion of division and control is far more damaging than just alienating a workforce. It can create Failure Demand, which in turn reduces an organisation's ability to overcome chaos, and increase throughput, through lower utilisation (see Chapter 6). The ideologies that drive greater control can increase fragmentation, the very thing that countless integration initiatives are seeking to overcome. For true integration, to defragment and create unity of effort, we argue systems, services and professionals need to question their work more fundamentally. The principles to overcome Failure Demand explored in this domain of Defragmenting to Integrate will help in that questioning as new models of care are considered. This will help avoid just addressing symptoms of system challenges, and help to address the root causes – the ideologies that shape our systems of care in the first place.

It would be fallacious to expect our systems to let go of these ideas overnight, or even in the near to medium term, but they can meaningfully explore them and challenge their own assumptions through prototyping. This is different to piloting, that of expecting a binary good/bad answer, but rather an iterative process designed to learn and refine an innovation, and the reinforcing assumptions behind the system in equal measure. This requires our leaders to participate rather than instruct. Systems of governance, hierarchy, measurement and mandate (role definition) should be challenged in equal measure along with the actual service structure and organisation.

It would also be easy to completely demonise these ideologies and their manifestation in healthcare systems. In the past these ideologies have brought real benefit – but perhaps now it is the time to bring them to the forefront and reflect upon them wholeheartedly. In parts of industry just this has happened. The emergence of Lean Thinking (Jones & Womack, 2003) was a response in industry to the forces described in this chapter. While many who try and replicate Lean in healthcare concentrate on the highly visible themes of Waste, Flow and Pull – and the associated highly enticing tools such as workplace organisation (5S) and process mapping, few really understand the first key principle, that of taking time to understand value in the first place, understanding core purpose and the relentless pursuit of delivering it. In other words, consider if you are doing the right work in the first place, otherwise you run the risk of making the wrong work efficient.

The same point is made in the works of Deming, whose thinking underpins much of what is codified in Lean Thinking. His teaching and subsequent publications *Out of Crisis* (Deming, 2000) and *The New Economics* (Deming, 2018) are a reflection and response to the same ideologies that, as discussed in Chapters 2 and 3, have influenced some of the leading healthcare thinkers of our time, such as Brent James, founder of Intermountain Healthcare's internationally renowned work on quality, and Don Berwick, former president and CEO of the Institute for Healthcare Improvement and advisor to the Obama administration. Yet, as with Lean Thinking, much of the core teaching has not been adopted widely, in particular the notion of reflecting upon the Theory of Knowledge, the ideologies that shape our systems of work. This is perhaps why the fragmentation persists and why the principles we propose to achieve integration are important – as they bridge the gap towards the practical application in healthcare.

As discussed, this is a question of balance where at the moment, in 2023 in the English NHS and in other systems, there is very little nuance or balance in our systems of operational management – perpetuated by a sense of crisis. Again, a deep questioning of the work and assumptions, using the methods, amongst others, of understanding of variation discussed in Chapter 4, detailed in this and subsequent chapters, go a long way to understanding when work needs a different approach and how to begin to achieve that. To overcome the fragmentation in our systems of care, for true integration, we should look to simplify, not just to consolidate or widen control and communication. We should work to avoid referring or defer-ring wherever possible, and do this by challenging the traditional role boundaries. In many settings this requires the letting go of the self-defeating temptation for further control, and the perspective needs to change from one of top-down atomi-sation and division of the work, to one of end-to-end understanding and minimal de-coupling caused by transitions. To do this we need to consider assessments as something for knowledge creation, not gatekeeping, and lastly work on mecha-nisms to help complexity to be held safely and effectively at lower levels.

Acknowledgements

We would like to thank Professor Becky Malby and Paul Jansen for their contribu-tion in helping to shape our thoughts on the impact of ideology, hierarchy and self-directed team working.

Notes

1   The thinking of Richard Davis on this subject of the impact of labelling needs, in his text *Responsibility and Public Service* (Davis, 2016), is enlightening.
2   The work of Hillary Cottam explores in great depth the importance of relation-ships in a functioning and effective welfare state (Cottam, 2018).

References

BMJ. 1972. Integrated hospital services – Letter to the editor. *British Medical Journal*, 1(5792): 115.
BMJ. 2020. *Opinion – Why Are So Many Doctors Quitting the NHS?* https://blogs.bmj.com/bmj/2020/02/06/why-are-so-many-doctors-quitting-the-nhs/
Britnell, M. 2015. *In Search of the Perfect Health System*. Palgrave Macmillan.
Commonwealth Fund. 2016. *Brazil's Family Health Strategy: Using Community Health Workers to Provide Primary Care*. www.commonwealthfund.org/publications/case-study/2016/dec/brazils-family-health-strategy-using-community-health-care-workers
Cottam, H. 2018. *Radical Help*. Virago Press.
Dansen, P. 2011. Challenges and opportunities facing medical education. *Transactions of the American Clinical and Climatological Association*, 122: 48–58.
Davis, R. 2016. *Responsibility in Public Services*. Triarchy Press.
Deming, W.E. 2018. *The New Economics* (3rd edn). The MIT Press.
Deming, W.E. 2000. *Out of Crisis*. MIT Press.

Downham, N. 2020. *Understanding the Work of Healthcare*. https://www.cressbrookltd. co.uk/understandingtheworkofhealthcare/

Gawande, A. 2014. *BBC Radio 4 – The Reith Lectures*. www.bbc.co.uk/programmes/ b04sv1s5

Ham, C. and Curry, N. 2011. *Integrated Care – What Is It? Does It Work? What Does It Mean for the NHS?* www.kingsfund.org.uk/sites/default/files/field/field_publication_ file/integrated-care-summary-chris-ham-sep11.pdf

Healthcare, I. 2018. *LSBU Health Services Innovation Lab Quality Improvement Study Tour* (Presentation, Salt Lake City, Utah, 12th February).

HM Government. 2017. *More Undergraduate Medical Education Places*. www.gov.uk/ government/news/more-undergraduate-medical-education-places

Intermountain Healthcare. 2016. *Integrated Team-Based Care Study Results in Improving Health Care Quality, Use and Costs*. https://intermountainhealthcare.org/blogs/ topics/research/2016/08/new-jama-study/

Jansen, P. 2019. *The Buurtzorg Back Office*. www.buurtzorg.org.uk/the-buurtzorg- back-office-by-paul-jansen/

Jansen, P. 2023. *Integrated Community Nursing Buurtzorg Model*. Guest Lecture, PCN Leadership Programme, Health Systems Innovation Lab, London South Bank University, 2nd February 2023.

Jenkins, S. 2022. Professions, heal yourself – only you can make the public sector better value for money. *The Guardian*, 22nd November.

Jones, D. and Womack, J. 2003. *Lean Thinking* (1st edn). Simon & Schuster UK Ltd.

Juran, J.M. 1989. *Juran on Leadership for Quality – An Executive Handbook*. Free Press.

Juran – Attain Partners. 2019. *Pareto Principle (80/20 Rule) & Pareto Analysis Guide*. www.juran.com/blog/a-guide-to-the-pareto-principle-80-20-rule-pareto-analysis/

Kennedy, C. 2007. *Guide to Management Gurus* (4th edn). Random House.

King's Fund. 2022. *Key Facts and Figures about the NHS*. www.kingsfund.org.uk/ audio-video/key-facts-figures-nhs

Lawrence, P. and Lorsch, J. 1967. New management job: The integrator. *Harvard Business Review – The Magazine*, November.

Monitor. 2015. *Integrated Care*. Monitor.

NHS Health Careers. n.d. *Explore Roles*. www.healthcareers.nhs.uk/explore-roles/ explore-roles

Seddon, J. 2005. *Freedom from Command and Control* (2nd edn). Vanguard Education Ltd.

Smith, A. 1776. *An Inquiry into the Nature of the Wealth of Nations*. Strahan and Cadell.

Weber, M. 2013. *Economy and Society* (Vol. 2). Translation based on 4th edition 1956 edn by Fischoff et al. University of California Press.

Wickens, P. 1998. *The Ascendant Organisation*. Palgrave Macmillan.

9

Avoiding the Specialist, Generalist and Citizen Muddle

The previous chapter, discussed the consequences of the intentional division of work through the principles of division of labour and bureaucratic design. We discussed that from certain perspectives the division of the work can deliver productivity gains, especially locally. We also explored where it can cause issues of fragmentation and the problems of quality that follow. In these discussions we used the wider definition of quality from the Institute of Medicine to include efficiency and effectiveness in addition to experience, safety and equity (Institute of Medicine, 2001). By surfacing some of the ideological themes that often promote this division of work and fragmentation, we proposed a series of design principles, principles of quality thinking, to use when designing and improving systems of work in order to avoid these problems. These were principles of Defragmenting to Integrate.

Framing

In this chapter we look at the muddle that plays out daily in our predominantly hierarchical models of care – the Specialist, Generalist and Citizen Muddle. At the end of Chapter 6, we introduced the idea as one of four potential sources of Failure Demand. It describes the muddle characterised by specialist work being done by generalists, generalist work being done by specialists and work being done by both that should be the domain of citizens and communities. In other words, work being done in the wrong settings and by the wrong people and often at the wrong time – usually too late. We argue this muddle risks a sub-optimum response to need and is often a source of Failure Demand created by, in no small part, avoidable transitions of care (see Chapters 6 and 8 for an explanation of how transitions can create Failure Demand).

This muddle can be found in the relationships between all parts of the NHS system of care and other developed health systems. Starting from the perspective of secondary care, the NHS Getting It Right First Time (GIRFT) programme, which aims to reduce unwarranted variation in hospitals in the English NHS, found inappropriate settings and referrals a major issue in a number of different disciplines. For example, in Ear, Nose and Throat departments, a significant proportion of hospitals had high levels of admissions at weekends where the admission was not followed by a dominant (surgical) procedure. This suggests that patients were being admitted to specialist settings which potentially could have been avoided (GIRFT, 2019a). Illustrating issues in the opposite direction, in Spinal Surgery the GIRFT team found a significant number of spinal procedures, regarded as specialist, being undertaken by non-specialist units (GIRFT, 2019b). Moving to Oral and Maxillofacial surgery, a significant proportion of high volume dentoalveolar surgery carried out in secondary care specialist settings was found to be more suited to intermediary or primary care dental settings (GIRFT, 2018). In Gynaecology services, which are typically under huge pressure, there were valuable opportunities for more conservative self-managed treatment and treatment supported by intermediate care rather than specialist settings (GIRFT, 2021b). As a final example, similar suggestions were made in Geriatric Medicine, e.g. large numbers of admissions of frail elderly people who would be better cared for at home or with community support if earlier assessments could be made (GIRFT, 2021a). In all these disciplines the messages were similar. Inappropriate settings and referrals led to issues such as delays, avoidable admissions, re-admissions and the avoidable use of specialist input.

Perhaps the oldest, most entrenched and dominant muddle in our health system is the relationship between primary and secondary care. This is as old as organised healthcare itself. General Practitioners (GPs) and other community care professionals have for years complained that patients are discharged too early from hospital – either because they are medically unfit or because they lack a care package or other form of support. From the other perspective, hospital clinicians have complained about GPs referring people inappropriately for specialist assessment or to emergency settings. Within GP practices themselves, the generalist and specialist muddle continues. Audits of GP appointments, by GPs themselves, have found significant proportions of appointments were more suited to more junior clinicians, non-clinicians and community services such as pharmacists (NHS England, 2015).

The muddle also plays out in different ways beyond the tension between primary and secondary care. It is also visible between tertiary centres and less specialist hospitals. As mentioned in Chapter 6, the Royal College of Paediatrics and Child Health found that 33% of patients in Paediatric Intensive Care Units could be in more local, less specialist, High Dependency Units (Royal College of Paediatrics and Child Health, 2018). This means a third of patients were unnecessarily taking up valuable capacity in one of the most expensive settings in any healthcare setting. It also has the consequence of adding additional travel, during times of immense worry, for some families as specialist unit beds may be a considerable distance away.

Even within single disciplines there is complexity in this muddle. A joint report on Paediatric Interventional Radiology (PIR), by the Royal College of Paediatrics and Child Health and the Royal College of Radiologists, found that some procedures were so specialist they need to be carried out by specialist Paediatric Radiologists, and that small and medium-sized hospitals are unlikely to have enough volume to justify and support PIR. Conversely, it was also found that that many PIR procedures could also be performed by appropriately trained non-radiologists (The Royal College of Radiologists, 2010). This suggests the two-way nature of untangling the muddle. It is not just a case of avoiding unnecessary use of specialists, but also the case that in some instances systems need to use them more.

At the most specialised end of specialisms there can often be single centre specialisms with just one unit in the country. This can provide benefits of consolidating rare expertise and providing the necessary volumes of cases, but it can also pose unique challenges in terms of governance and scrutiny. The ongoing scandal involving the Gender Identity Development Service at the Tavistock Institute in London is exposing alleged deficiencies in systems of internal oversight and whistleblowing (Cooke, 2021). While reports question internal process, another perspective could be the limited external network and professional inter-centre working caused by single centre specialism. This lack of external network could potentially create echo chambers and reduce the effectiveness of external checks and balances.

Design Principles to Avoid the Specialist, Generalist and Citizen Muddle

In this chapter we will be exploring the causes of this muddle, and also introduce and discuss a set of design principles that we argue are important in designing services to avoid it. These are detailed in summary in Figure 9.1.

- Generalists valued as much as specialists
- Specialists support (consult in) generalists (or whoever holds the relationship with the patient) wherever appropriate
- Seek to avoid referring and deferring – maximum subsidiarity
- The professions promote broadening of responsibilities towards 'doing hat matters'
- Frameworks and governance support professionals to do a wider span of activities
- Mechanisms in place to keep work in ore general/non-specialist settings wherever possible

---

Figure 9.1   Specialist, generalist and citizen muddle

As discussed in Chapter 8, the NHS has been designed with hierarchy and specialism as guiding principles. One of the prominent themes in this chapter is the inappropriate use of these specialist structures, settings and professionals within.

This, to a large degree, is because specialists are like powerful magnets in our care systems; work gravitates to specialists if left unchecked – appropriate or not. Perhaps driven by fear of litigation, staffing, demand pressures and even patient expectations, many care decisions and interventions are deferred and referred to specialists and specialist centres. Yet as discussed in the beginning of this chapter, the use of these most expensive of resources can potentially be avoided; freeing up valuable capacity for those who do need it.

As with most of this book, we are talking here about tensions rather than absolutes. It is a question of balance. We propose that the balance can be better achieved with these design principles during periods of service configuration, improvement and review. Without a set of visible design principles to reflect against, the gravitation towards the specialist will always prevail – regardless of how appropriate their use is – or not.

Value the Generalist

Leading healthcare thinkers such as Don Berwick,[1] founding CEO of the Institute for Healthcare Improvement, and John Wennberg, Director Emeritus at the Dartford Institute for Health Policy and Clinical Practice, have highlighted this natural gravitation towards specialist settings in their thinking on the problems facing established healthcare systems such as those in the USA and in the UK. Berwick, in a high-profile speech to leaders of the English NHS, advised the NHS to "avoid supply driven care like the plague" (Berwick, 2008, p. 214). In supply driven care, Berwick is referring to the supply of hospital, or specialist care. He argues that if you plan your system on creating supply of such capacity, this capacity will always be used – appropriately or not. This illustrates the natural gravitation towards specialists and specialist settings we describe. Foreshadowing the danger he sees in the English NHS potentially following the US healthcare system down a route of private providers, he is reflecting on the amplification of this natural gravitation by market forces. If you mix supply driven care with commercial provision of that supply, the emphasis will always be on the very high utilisation of that supply to ensure commercial return, regardless of whether more appropriate settings or models are available. This is perhaps a large part of the reason the US healthcare system is the most expensive in the world, with arguably some of the worst population level outcomes (Commonwealth Fund, 2020). John Wennberg, a leading thinker on unwarranted variation in healthcare, made the same point in his pivotal writing on unwarranted variation driven by supply sensitive care (Wennberg, 2002). As we discussed in Chapter 4, Wennberg argues that use of healthcare facilities, including their doctors, is often not driven by medical theory or evidence, but by their availability – or their supply. Put simply, the more supply, the more utilisation. This is why we have to be mindful of the phenomenon of supply driven utilisation as it is one of the reasons for the gravitational pull towards specialist settings.

The opposite of a specialist in many systems is the generalist. When it comes to avoiding Failure Demand caused by fragmentation, generalists are part of the solution as they not only allow a system to hold care in less specialist settings, but they also reduce transitions of care. A highly skilled generalist, with the right support, can "hold" a valuable proportion of cases and resolve them without requiring transitions to specialists. This not only protects valuable specialist capacity, but also reduces the risk of Failure Demand.

Of course, at this point we need to make clear that specialism continues to matter and be central to our systems of care. For example it has been established that there are better outcomes for emergency patients in major trauma centres (Moran et al., 2018) rather than in smaller less specialist hospitals (NHS England, 2018b). Another example of the need for further specialism, which illustrates that we must continually review our services, can be found in stroke services. In stroke services the recent move to mechanical thrombectomy offers better outcomes to patients (NHS England, 2018a) but it is extremely time sensitive and requires more specialist input than previous interventions. This means the provision of the required 24 hour services cannot happen without pooling of resources and volume of patients – thus necessitating a specialist hub and spoke, or regionalised specialist centre, model. In primary care similar patterns can be found. Evidence suggests that for accurate interpretation of spirometry, vital for accurate diagnosis of chronic obstructive pulmonary disease (COPD), and also to reduce the often-common levels of COPD under-diagnosis, a specialist diagnostic hub model can improve quality (Hodges, 2021). This mirrors our own practical experience of improving spirometry, where the interpretation of spirometry requires sufficient volume and supervision in order for a clinician to maintain competency – something that was not always possible with a single practice approach.

Referrals to specialist assessment will always be a key feature of our system, especially with the advancement of medical knowledge and capability – but they need to be appropriate, rather than being driven by gravitational forces such as defensive medicine, public expectation and systemic devaluation of the role of generalists. Given the volumes of referrals between more generalist and specialist clinicians, even relatively small percentages of inappropriate settings can add up to huge absolute numbers and can make the difference between stable and overloaded systems.

With this gravitation towards specialism, the value of generalists has been eroded over time. Through our lens of Failure Demand, generalists such as GPs, or in secondary care roles such as general medicine doctors and geriatricians, help provide and maintain care without Failure Demand potentially triggering transitions to further specialisms. This is highlighted by the Royal College of General Practitioners in detailing one of the many roles of GPs as "risk managers that recognise that not all symptomatology requires investigation, referral or treatment" (Royal College of

General Practitioners, 2018). We argue that without sufficient generalists, at all levels, our systems of care will become more fragmented and more difficult to integrate.

Specialists Support Generalists, Wherever Appropriate – Maximum Subsidiarity

Many of the transitions between generalists and specialists, including between more and less specialist clinicians, are to access specialist opinion and advice. The traditional approach to getting that advice being a referral – triggering a transition. But this is not the only way generalists can get specialist input. By organising so that generalists are supported in a different way by specialists, these transitions can potentially be avoided.

As we touched on in Chapter 8, the much-celebrated Intermountain Mental Health pathway achieves just this. Enabled by decision-support algorithms, family practitioners are helped to hold patients to a greater extent in order to avoid the overuse of specialist settings (Healthcare, 2018; Intermountain Healthcare, 2016). They are provided access to different types of mental health specialists who consult into the family practitioner as well as being available to refer to if appropriate.

Illustrating how this principle can apply in different parts of health and social care systems, the promising "no wrong door" prototyping in Hastings and St Leonards in the UK is focused on enabling first line services, in this case in the voluntary sector such as food banks, to provide advice for common queries that would usually require a referral or visit to the more specialist Citizens Advice Bureau (CAB). The key points are that the first line service often has the relationship and thus the trust of the person needing the help and also a significant proportion of queries that go to CAB are relatively simple to resolve with quite modest training and information (NHS Sussex ICS and Health Systems Innovation Lab LSBU, 2023).

Another example of moves towards new models where specialists offer greater support to generalists can be found in Paediatrics. In North West London, led by Consultant Paediatrician Dr Tom Holliday, there are prototypes of monthly joint GP/Paediatric clinics in primary care combined with virtual MDT meetings. Specialist paediatricians consult alongside GPs. These monthly child health hubs have proven to reduce Paediatric referrals from general practice, shorten the time it takes children to receive the support they need, and reduce the system cost of providing children with the care they need. They also create better ongoing relationships with generalists, serve to upskill the generalists further and have been warmly received by children and parents. The team behind the work stress that the work is not process improvement, but a change to the traditional ways of organising regarding specialists and generalists. The team also highlight one of the structural challenges: the implications of loss of revenue for some of the stakeholders due to the change in model (Holliday, 2023).

System and speciality leaders should be cognisant of the pros and cons of different structures that provide specialist input into clinical practice and decisions. Without this consideration we risk sleepwalking into mirroring the age-old structures that we have always wrestled with. An example of this is the new structures proposed by the Primary Care Diabetes Society (PCDS) in the NHS, aimed at improving prevention and management of type 2 diabetes against the backdrop of greatly increasing demand and complexity of patients. One of the number of recommendations is to create a new tier in the structure – where a specialist (tier 2) type 2 diabetes team is created at the level of the Primary Care Network (PCN – typically a group of general practices that work together on a footprint of 30,000–50,000 patients). The proposal is the specialist team take on patients who are unable to be managed at practice level (tier 1) or are not meeting treatment targets (Primary Care Diabetes Association, 2021). While this new structure brings welcome further capability for general practice, it illustrates a proliferation of further levels of specialism. In this model the specialist team is positioned in a traditional manner to hold their own case load. Through the lens of Failure Demand, this creates a new transition of care and potential micro queues and silos within the PCN. An alternative could be that the specialist team are focused on supporting the practices (tier 1) to hold the patients. This would ensure provision of advice, potentially consulting into the tier 1 clinicians in multi-disciplinary team consultations, building skills and confidence, creating systems of decision support and avoiding the deskilling of tier 1 clinicians. In highlighting this alternative way of organising, we are not dismissing the originally proposed structure, but rather are suggesting that we need to ensure the pros and cons of introducing more tiers of specialism are at the front of mind when considering such structures.

Catalysed by the COVID-19 pandemic starting in 2020, there have been moves by secondary care specialities to be more accessible to generalist settings, such as general practice, with the aim of avoiding referrals. A common move is for specialities to provide single points of access for general practitioners to contact with queries about patients. Our experience is that geriatric, endocrine and renal medicine are some of the more progressive specialties in this manner. Other models feature monitored email addresses which specialists monitor as part of their job plans. These moves are obviously welcomed and are often touted as innovations – although many general practitioners will remember it was not that long ago that general practitioners could phone specialists directly if they felt that a bit of advice could avoid a referral into a specialist setting. The provision of support for more generalist settings can be further enabled by adoption of synchronous and asynchronous digital channels and potentially through artificial intelligence enabled decision support tools.

The direction of travel here is towards maximum subsidiarity – that is designing and organising to ensure the holding of work at the lowest safe and effective level. This is not a new idea and is a principle that has been at the heart of first principles quality thinking for decades – as detailed by Joseph Juran,[2] one of the big three quality thinkers of our time, in his writing on maximum delegation to the workforce (Juran, 1989). An example of the importance high-performance health systems place on this can be found in the much-studied Southcentral Foundation NUKA system of care in Alaska – where all staff are encouraged to work at the "top of their licence" and physicians who fail to delegate their work are not compensated for their resulting longer hours (Baker & Denis, 2011). In the NHS there are moves towards this type of model, although without the incentives to delegate, with the establishing of neighbourhood teams to enable closer working between acute, intermediate and community providers. As usual, it is what matters beneath the title that will judge whether this is successful. If these moves towards greater integration are implemented with maximum subsidiarity in mind, with the resulting changes in the relationships between specialists and generalists we have discussed in this chapter, then they offer a chance for genuine transformation of care. While we talk about this in terms of structure, perhaps the key enabler is supporting the humans at the centre of our structures – the patients, their families/carers and professionals. Less specialist and/or more junior clinicians, for example, will not hold work at the lowest possible level without feeling safe and proficient in doing so. To enable this the human system of work needs to change – tackling issues such as real and perceived risk of litigation, issues of accountability and access to support. These issues are discussed in detail in Chapter 10.

Framework and Governance to Support Professionals to Do a Wider Span of Activities

The traditional approach to planning roles and work is to ensure clarity of role, role boundaries and responsibility. To ensure everyone can understand which professional is responsible for what, and so that the individual professional understands exactly what it is they are responsible for – and also what they are not. The idea being that this makes things easier to manage. These highly defined roles are documented in the forms of job descriptions and are often supported by highly defined standard operating procedure and policy. This definition of role is generally done by someone senior, for execution by someone more junior.

Unfortunately, as we have learned in previous chapters, the difficulty in this lies in the fact that a collection of highly defined roles doesn't automatically operate as a harmonious collective whole. It is very likely to result in boundaries, problematic transitions between professionals and professionals retreating into their role or team silos at times of great pressure – severe pressure being something most professionals are constantly under in the current state of many healthcare systems. As professionals retreat into their silos and concentrate on their defined role – their "bit" – it is quite possible for a complex patient to move between professionals, even within multi-disciplinary team structures, and no one take effective responsibility for them. This role definition can lead to an illusion of accountability and control, but in reality there is very little of either.

The counter to this problem of tightly defined roles is to design roles with deliberate overlap (Jansen, 2023). This is horizontal overlap – between peers – and also vertical overlap between more senior and junior, or generalist and more specialist professionals. To achieve this overlap a broadening of skillset and skill mix is required. The overlap avoids a valuable proportion of the Failure Demand caused by the handoffs and transitions we discussed in Chapters 6 and 8. It also removes the silos and encourages collaboration. In the English NHS, the vertical element of this systemic broadening of responsibilities or skill mix is beginning to gain traction and be recognised as part of the mix of reforms required to improve productivity (Horton et al., 2021).

Perhaps the most radical visualisation of this idea can be found in Frederic Laloux's typology of organisational models, in his thinking on leading edge "Teal" organisations and in particular self-managing teams. His writing pulls on the example of the highly successful Buurtzorg Nursing model we have discussed previously. Who better to define roles than those closest to the work – a self-managing team themselves – a process he describes as role trading (Laloux, 2014).

Ultimately perhaps the biggest barrier to the introduction of new broader roles or changing/challenging traditional role boundaries is one of governance and regulation (Commonwealth Fund, 2016; Jansen, 2023). Broader, overlapping roles just don't fit easily in existing systems that predominantly pursue individual, rather than collective, accountability. Collective accountability is one of the key requirements of healthcare systems which seek to improve their quality and reliability, where they are currently held back by traditional systems of governance (Britnell, 2015).

Do We Control Outcomes?

For many of the greatest challenges that face health services in developed and many developing economies, it can be argued it is not health services themselves that control outcomes. In the UK at least, health services typically adopt a paternalistic relationship with patients – with the expectation that the professional is there to take responsibility and "fix" the patient. This expectation is deeply seated in both the public and professional psyche. The highest proportion of the major health conditions that form much of the challenges facing health systems, such as many cancers, cardiovascular disease, stroke, diabetes and respiratory disease, are greatly influenced by patients themselves and their social and environmental context. In a useful summary of the social determinants, the King's Fund, while listing three separate studies, list the healthcare determinants as only being between 15% and 45% of the determinants of someone's health outcomes (The King's Fund, 2012).

While we discuss this in greater detail in Chapter 11, the acceptance of the impact of the social determinants poses a huge challenge to the focus of healthcare systems and those who work within them. Returning to the Southcentral Foundation's NUKA model of care, with its internationally recognised achievements, it is worth noting that it is to a great extent based on this premise. That for much of care, it is not health services in any traditional sense that control outcomes with patients. The Southcentral Foundation build their system on the understanding that for the majority of low- and medium-complexity work, it is patients and their families who control outcomes (Anderson-Wallace, 2014; Collins, 2015). For example, take a pressing example from the English NHS – that of type 2 diabetes. It is the person and their context, which is often intertwined with their family unit, that controls many of the outcomes. Where a person lives and what access they have to healthy ingredients can have a massive impact. What patterns and rituals their family and social network have around mealtimes and food consumption will also have a considerable influence on their ability to follow a diet. The nature of a person's employment will affect their ability to exercise as will access to safe recreational space. Southcentral build their system on the view that the person-in-context remains dominant to the point where more acute intervention is required. Because they believe that for low and medium complexity it is the person-in-context that controls outcomes, they organise in a way that supports this. This includes working with families, with social and cultural context firmly in mind.

This leads us to the third part of our muddle – the citizen. In addition to the muddle between specialists and generalists, health services often intervene where communities and their citizens are much better placed to do so. If we view our patients with a paternalistic, deficit mindset, we will continue along the traditional path of seeking to understand "what is making people ill?" and providing solutions. An asset-based mindset instead starts with the question "what makes us healthy?" (Rippon & Hopkins, 2015). Starting with this question leads us to the social and environmental determinants we discussed earlier in this chapter. The Asset Based Health Enquiry by the Health System's Innovation Lab at London South Bank University strongly suggests that communities are often more capable at helping themselves, helping their citizens, than professionals and leaders often assume; that health services should concentrate more on connecting citizens with communities and the volunteer and community network within them (Malby et al., 2019). Returning to the type 2 diabetes example, a patient can have five to ten scheduled and unscheduled interactions with health services in a year – leaving perhaps 355 days a year where they don't have any support or contact. In this time, it is the patient who controls the outcomes and it is here where self-management and peer-enabled support should be focused.

The potential of self and community management is not just focused on the high-volume chronic conditions. Self-management is rapidly increasing alongside the advances in digital technology and medical devices. Traditionally complex inpatient interventions can now be self-managed. For example, home dialysis technology now allows for dialysis at home for many patients (NHS Kidney Care, 2010). Oncology services can now be provided in the community much closer to patients (University Hospitals Bristol and Weston NHS Foundation Trust, 2021) and everyday technologies such as smart phones are opening up possibilities to move a host of diagnostic monitoring activities into the hands of the patient.

The Professions Promote Broadening of Responsibilities Towards "Doing What Matters"

A key enabler for the patient to be more prominent and effective in their own care is professionals recalibrating the intention and focus of their consultations, especially those such as annual reviews and diagnosis of long-term conditions. In a traditional review consultation, the terminology and goal setting is often clinical. On top of this the patient is, as described by Simon Eaton, a consultant diabetologist at Northumbria Healthcare NHS Foundation Trust in the UK, often trying to deal with the "bewildering risk progression or complications; the relentless lifestyle and personal changes they are encouraged to make to avoid these; the complexity of multiple conditions and polypharmacy, as well as the emotional and social implications of each of these to the person and their families" (Eaton, 2016, p.128). The risk, as described by Eaton, is that faced with passive and unsurprisingly poorly engaged patients, clinicians may revert to a "fix it" mentality. As we have discussed, this temptation to assume a paternalistic relationship with a person can be amplified by professional ideology and also by expectations from people themselves. This is something Atul Gawande describes, in his excellent BBC Reith Lectures on the future of medicine, as health systems being *fooled by penicillin*. He refers to the expectations built up in the 20th century that we would be able to develop further easy injections to cure cancers, heart disease and stroke (Gawande, 2014). Our observations from talking to clinicians is that this expectation of an easy fix to conditions has propagated into the views of many patients. Considering this backdrop, it is perhaps unsurprising that for conditions such as type 1 diabetes in England, which involves the coordination of primary, intermediate and secondary care touch points, the number of patients achieving all three of the diabetes treatment targets,[3] which represent a useful and repeatable proxy for good outcomes, was just 21.5% of diagnosed patients in 2021 (NHS Digital, 2022).

An example of systemically overcoming these issues and challenging these poor outcomes is the Year of Care Approach. Developed by the Department of Health in the UK, it is a person-centred care approach that is sometimes referred to as personalised care planning. The approach broadens the scope of consultations towards doing "what matters" in partnership with patients. It focuses consultations on what matters for the patient and tries to avoid the complexity, bewilderment and passivity previously described. This has been shown to result in improvements in indicators of psychological and physical health and people's ability to self-manage (Coutier et al., 2015). It does this with several core principles (Eaton, 2016): shared power and partnership, acknowledging the assets each party brings (the patient being the expert in their life and context) and a biopsychosocial approach.[4] To enable this reorientation of focus and relationship, changes to pathways, administration, communication and diagnostics processes (Year of Care Partnerships, n.d.) are required in order to maximise generative and patient-centred dialogue time with the patient.

The core message in this example is for health services, and their professionals, to pause and consider if their consultations are focused on doing what matters, in a way that matters for patients, or whether they are just focused on what fits organisationally or ideologically.

Conclusions

This domain of Failure Demand, the Specialist, Generalist, and Citizen Muddle, provides the second of our lenses to question the work – focused on who is best placed to do the work and in what setting. The untangling of this muddle offers great opportunity for quality improvement, including efficiency, at not only health provider level but at the level of health system. We argue that the detangling of this muddle can be helped by the principles of maximum subsidiarity, greater support of generalists, more holistic support of patients, challenging of traditional role boundaries and greater collective rather than individual accountability. This is all supported by recalibrating interactions with patients to ensure they are focused on what matters to patients in a language that matters – failure to achieve this risks further propagating paternal and passive relationships with patients.

We believe the design principles we have identified require constant focus. That some of the forces that cause this muddle, especially that of the pull of specialism, are like gravity. Left unchecked, the muddle will likely re-establish itself even after deliberate attempts to avoid it. Technological, clinical and psychosocial advancements mean that systems will consistently and frequently need to check assumptions on where work is done, and who it is best done by. This can mean more specialism, but in many cases it will mean the opposite. Regardless of the direction of travel, the core competence our services need to excel at is one of letting go. This means not only letting go of work, but also letting go of funding and structures associated with certain types of work, in order to enable work to be done elsewhere.

Finally, it is worth noting that in this second of our Principles to Avoid Failure Demand domain chapters, you will begin to have noticed the links between the other three domain chapters. Some of the same causes surface in more than one of them and the resulting design principles are often inter-related. As with everything in the systemic improvement of quality this is an example of the impossibility of neat solutions and frameworks. We have split this discussion into domains to aid discussion and to provide a more effective heuristic for often busy leaders. But as they are explored, we encourage them to be viewed as a whole.

Acknowledgements

We would like to thank Dr Iolanthe Fowler and Dr Tom Holliday for sharing their expertise and thinking in discussions that have shaped this chapter.

Notes

1 See Chapter 2 for more detail on Don Berwick's influential thinking on quality in healthcare.
2 The other two being W. Edwards Deming and Philip Crosby.
3 HBA1c ≤ 58mmol/mol, BP ≤ 140/80, people within CVD prevention group – receiving statins.
4 A principle we explore in depth in Chapter 11.

References

Anderson-Wallace, M. 2014. *Understanding NUKA – A Proposal for Systemic Learning.* Centre for Innovation and Health Management, The University of Leeds.

Baker, G.R. and Denis, J.-L. 2011. *A Comparative Study of Three Transformative Health-care Systems: Lessons for Canada.* Canadian Health Services Research Foundation.

Berwick, D. 2008. A transatlantic review of the NHS at 60. *BMJ,* 337: 212. www.bmj.com/bmj/section-pdf/186530?path=/bmj/337/7663/Analysis.full.pdf

Britnell, M. 2015. *In Search of the Perfect Health System.* Palgrave Macmillan.

Collins, B. 2015. *Intentional Whole Systems Health System Redesign: Southcentral Foundation's NUKA System of Care.* The King's Fund.

Commonwealth Fund. 2016. *Brazil's Family Health Strategy: Using Community Health Workers to Provide Primary Care.* www.commonwealthfund.org/publications/case-study/2016/dec/brazils-family-health-strategy-using-community-health-care-workers

Commonwealth Fund. 2020. *US Health Care from a Global Perspective, 2019: Higher Spending, Worse Outcomes.* The Commonwealth Fund.

Cooke, R. 2021. Tavistock Trust Whistleblower David Bell "I believed I was doing the right thing". *The Guardian,* 2nd May.

Coulter, A., Entwistle, V., Eccles, A., Ryan, S., Sheppard, S. and Perera, P. 2015. *Personalised Care Planning for Adults with Chronic or Long-Term Health Conditions.* Cochrane Library, Wiley.

Eaton, S. 2016. Delivering person-centred care in long-term conditions. *Future Hospital, Journal Royal College of Physicians*, 3(2): 128–131.

Gawande, A. 2014. *BBC Radio 4 – The Reith Lectures*. www.bbc.co.uk/programmes/b04sv1s5

GIRFT – Getting It Right First Time. 2018. *Oral and Maxillofacial Surgery GIRFT National Programme Speciality Report*. NHS.

GIRFT – Getting It Right First Time. 2019a. *Ear, Nose and Throat Surgery GIRFT Programme National Speciality Report*. NHS.

GIRFT – Getting It Right First Time. 2019b. *Spinal Services – GIRFT Programme National Speciality Report*. NHS.

GIRFT – Getting It Right First Time. 2021a. *Geriatric Medicine GIRFT National Programme National Programme Speciality Report*. NHS.

GIRFT – Getting It Right First Time. 2021b. *Maternity and Gynaecology GIRFT National Programme Speciality Report*. NHS.

Healthcare, I. 2018. *LSBU Health Services Innovation Lab Quality Improvement Study Tour* (Presentation, Salt Lake City, Utah, 12th February).

Hodges, R. 2021. *Lung Disease Diagnosis Pathway*. www.blf.org.uk/taskforce/about/our-diagnosis-working-group/lung-disease-diagnosis-pathway

Holliday, T. 2023. *Community Hospital Integrated Care*. London North West University Healthcare NHS Trust.

Horton, T., Mehay, A. and Warburton, W. 2021. *Agility: The Missing Ingredient for NHS Productivity*. The Health Foundation.

Institute of Medicine. 2001. *Crossing the Quality Chasm*. National Academies Press.

Intermountain Healthcare. 2016. *Integrated Team-Based Care Study Results in Improving Health Care Quality, Use and Costs*. https://intermountainhealthcare.org/blogs/topics/research/2016/08/new-jama-study/

Jansen, P. 2023. *Integrated Community Nursing Buurzorg Model*. Guest Lecture, PCN Leadership Programme, Health Systems Innovation Lab, London South Bank University, 2nd February 2023.

Juran, J.M. 1989. *Juran on Leadership for Quality – An Executive Handbook*. Free Press.

Laloux, F. 2014. *Reinventing Organisations*. Nelson Parker.

Malby, B., Boyle, D., Smith, S. and Ben Omar, S. 2019. *The Asset-Based Health Enquiry*. London South Bank University.

Moran, C., Lecky, F., Bouamra, O., Lawrence, T., Edwards, A., Woodford, M., Willett, K. and Coats, T. 2018. Changing the system – Major trauma patients and their outcomes in the NHS (England) 2008–17. *eClinical Medicine*, 2: 13–21.

NHS Digital. 2022. *National Diabetes Audit – Report 1: Care Processes and Treatment Targets 2020–21, Full Report*. https://digital.nhs.uk/data-and-information/publications/statistical/national-diabetes-audit/core-report-1-2020-21/care-processes-and-treatment-targets-national-summary-2015-2021

NHS England. 2015. *1 in 4 GP Appointments Potentially Avoidable*. www.england.nhs.uk/2015/10/gp-appointments/

NHS England. 2018a. *Clinical Commissioning Policy: Mechanical Thrombectomy for Acute Ischaemic Stroke (All Ages)*. NHS England.

NHS England. 2018b. *More Than 1,600 Extra Trauma Victims Alive Today Says Major New Study*. www.england.nhs.uk/2018/08/more-than-1600-extra-trauma-victims-alive-today-says-major-new-study/

NHS Kidney Care. 2010. *Improving Choice for Kidney Patients*. NHS.

NHS Sussex ICS and Health Systems Innovation Lab LSBU. 2023. *Universal Healthcare*. NHS.

Primary Care Diabetes Association. 2021. *Best Practice in the Delivery of Diabetes Care in the Primary Care Network*. Primary Care Diabetes Association.

Rippon, S. and Hopkins, T. 2015. *Heads, Hands and Heart: Asset-Based Approaches in Healthcare*. The Health Foundation.

Royal College of General Practitioners. 2018. Cited in "Divided we fall: Getting the best out of general practice". Nuffield Trust.

Royal College of Paediatrics and Child Health. 2018. *High Dependency Care for Children – Time to Move On*. www.rcpch.ac.uk/sites/default/files/2018-07/high_dependency_care_for_children_-_time_to_move_on.pdf

The King's Fund. 2012. *Broader Determinants of Health: Future Trends*. www.kingsfund.org.uk/projects/time-think-differently/trends-broader-determinants-health

The Royal College of Radiologists. 2010. *Improving Paediatric Interventional Radiology Services – An Intercollegiate Report*. The Royal College of Radiologists.

University Hospitals Bristol and Weston NHS Foundation Trust. 2021. *Chemotherapy in the Community*. University Hospitals Bristol and Weston NHS Foundation Trust.

Wennberg, J. 2002. Unwarranted variations in healthcare delivery: Implications for academic medical centres. *BMJ*, 325: 961–964.

Year of Care Partnerships. n.d. *The Year of Care House*. www.yearofcare.co.uk/year-care-house

10

Supporting Human Systems at Work

Framing

In this chapter we aim to explore principles to overcome Failure Demand under a domain that we have termed "Defensive Pressures". Our proposition here is that these pressures, which often go completely unnoticed - can drive unhelpful patterns of behaviour that significantly affect relationships and adversely influence the context of care. They detract significantly from the purpose of the work and eat up precious capacity - in short, they are extremely wasteful. They impact all the elements of quality we have been considering through our use of the Institute of Medicine's definition of quality - that of Safety, Effectiveness, Patient Centredness, Timeliness, Efficiency and Equity (Institute of Medicine, 2001). Worse still, they fracture - sometimes irrevocably - the crucial bond of trust between caregivers and citizens, not only at the level of service delivery but also in families, our communities and society more generally - the human cost is therefore immeasurable. In an environment of growing health inequity and unmet need in many communities, we need to promote the absolute opposite: creating greater clarity in expectations to build trust, and to use all the knowledge available in the therapeutic context to build more collaborative and equitable relations. Unless we do this, our current systems risk collapsing under a combination of growing cost pressures, unmet needs and rising levels of mistrust. Importantly, we also risk expunging the desperately needed humanity from our caring systems.

The good news is that evidence suggests that these pressures can be proactively addressed, but we first need to acknowledge their presence and understand their impact. There is also plenty of scope for intervention and development in these areas, although significant commitment to both philosophical and practical change is often needed.

Recognise the effect of the strange moral and psychological world of healthcare:

- Appreciate social systems defences against anxiety
- Promote the conditions for interpersonal risk and organisational health
- Institutional reflective practice and restorative approaches

---

Figure 10.1   Supporting human systems at work

In this chapter, we suggest four key areas for focus – see Figure 10.1. Firstly, we need to understand that providing healthcare is high risk work that takes place in a strange moral and psychological environment. Secondly, we need to understand the rise in defensive medicine and the associated medico-legal pressures that shape a great deal of daily practice and experience. These are both real and imagined, but either way the impacts are enormous. Thirdly, we need to address some key issues associated with the punitive culture in healthcare – both real and perceived. Finally, we want to draw attention to healthcare harm including our understanding of what constitutes safety improvement. Associated with this we need to address the notion of compounded harm that arises when the response to harm is poor quality. This involves understanding the need for both "healing" as well as "learning" when harm occurs. In this area, we also must explore the difficult and pervasive cultures of blame and shame, which are toxic for all concerned. Our argument is that insufficient attention has been given to this domain, and the systems of regulation and inspection that are intended to help, in practice, often seem to make the situation worse, not better.

Of course, while often marginalised in terms of real-world application, a focus on supporting human systems at work to improve quality is not new. As we discuss in detail in Chapter 2, W. Edwards Deming – the so-called "father of quality thinking" highlighted the critical influence of human psychology on achieving quality. This could be seen as Deming's direct reaction to the dominance of Taylorism as his theoretical position was predicated on the idea that best quality was achieved when individuals are respected, well-motivated and self-managed. Deming however still considered that managers could manipulate the system conditions through rational choice and design, and that this in turn leads to the desired changes in a logical and reliable manner – ironically this also included the introduction of self-management. The idea is contested by those who adopt a postmodern perspective, where a much messier appreciation of the emergent possibilities exists. Our own position is that whilst we recognise that leaders have a crucial role to play in creating the conditions of work, that unless we aim to engage all those with knowledge in the network of relationships that constitute "the work", then our picture will always be too narrow and unnecessarily partial. Recent evidence suggests that high degrees of collaboration across distributed networks of relationship are a major factor in successful quality improvement programmes (Burgess et al., 2022). A focus on the relational practices which support the development of the networks of relationships are crucial if we are to support the human system at work (Malby & Anderson-Wallace, 2016).

High-Risk Work and the Strange Moral and Psychological World of Healthcare

Healthcare is by its very nature a high-risk activity. This is generally well understood by those who work in healthcare but is a well-kept open secret beyond that. The stubbornly high levels of avoidable iatrogenic harm – that is harm caused by treatment, intentionally or not, in healthcare (WHO, 2019) – tends to come as a great surprise to most citizens, who quite understandably tend to think of healthcare as inherently safe. Clinicians engage in very intimate and often highly invasive work, both physically and psychologically. Much of what is done entirely legitimately in a healthcare context would in any other situation be seen as abusive or harmful. This inversion of the norm creates an unusual set of relationships and expectations, as well as a special bond of trust unlike most others in life, where those who need their help must trust others to act in their best interests, at times when they cannot do this for themselves (Shale, 2011). They often do this without any pre-existing relationship.

As sociologist Dan Chambliss eloquently points out:

> In the hospital it is the good people, not the bad, who take knives and cut people open; here the good stick others with needles and push fingers into rectums and vaginas, tubes into urethras, needles into the scalp of a baby; here the good, doing good, peel dead skin from a screaming burn victim's body and tell strangers to take off their clothes... The layperson's horrible fantasies here become the professional's stock in trade. (Chambliss, 1996)

This complex and often troubling moral world invisibly underpins the very recognisable everyday routines of healthcare delivery. These rituals and routines shape relationships in ways we have all become very accustomed to, and they are rarely questioned precisely because they appear so "normal" in the context. All of this is generally unnamed and unexplored, until something unexpected happens, at which point everyone's actions – including their moral positions – are called into question. Without active mitigation, the relational conditions created can easily become toxic. At best, this can lead to a lack of compassion and/or empathy between professionals and citizens – in both directions – and at worst, adversarial actions including neglect, abuse and litigation.

Social Systems Defence against Anxiety

Isabel Menzies-Lyth was a psychoanalyst and social researcher, who tried to develop a theory to understand how a lack of compassion could develop in caring organisations. She conducted ground-breaking research exploring the working conditions of nurses in an acute healthcare environment. The central thesis of what she discovered was that paradoxically, it was the motivation to care that could sometimes make health organisations uncaring. Menzies-Lyth (1960) identified a series of complex natural defences that as human beings we develop to protect us from the anxiety provoked by difficult and emotionally challenging work. In the healthcare setting, this often includes having close contact with people that are severely injured and whose bodily functions are often completely out of control. In the course of their daily work, healthcare workers meet illness, physical degeneration, disfigurement, psychological disturbance, emotional distress and death. Menzies-Lyth saw these experiences as "taboo" and concluded that performing this kind of work over time exposes those involved to a level of ambient anxiety. If over-exposed, she believed that the impact and consequences could be significant, if not catastrophic.

Menzies-Lyth argued that in response to this – as an act of protection – organisations try to prevent carers from becoming overwhelmed. Inadvertently, this frequently occurs by structuring the work in ways that enable – and occasionally even encourage – detachment from the patients as individuals. This can at first manifest in ways that seem quite benign. For instance, work becomes task-driven and is often carried out by several different people, making it uncommon for one staff member to follow a patient throughout their entire care journey. She noted that because both patients and staff were often transferred between care settings, all of them can be commodified and objectified through the language that is used to describe them. This often involves reducing the identity of staff members to their job roles and patients to their bed number or disease state.

Note that the points in the list in Figure 10.2 all serve to fragment care and create multiple handoffs – once of the sources of Failure Demand we explored in Chapters 6, 8 and 9.

As Jocelyn Cornwell, the founder and former Chief Executive of The Point of Care Foundation comments, "there is something deeply paradoxical about the dehumanising way in which patients are treated by organisations that are supposed to be people- and patient-centred". She posits that "it is because modern medicine is so successful technically, that patients' suffering seems to have been pushed from centre stage into the background" (Cornwell, 2021).

Examples of dehumanising, objectification and mechanistic approaches created as the social system's defence against anxiety:

- Splitting of caregiver relations – no continuity of care, shift arrangements, staff treated as moveable resources, task rather than person-centred care
- Depersonalizing and categorization of patients and staff – referring to "the med reg" – "the fractured NOF in bed 3"
- Failure to define fully who handles a patient's care leading to fragmentation and multiple hand-offs
- Delegation upwards of responsibility for task leading to alienation and mechanical delivery of care

Figure 10.2   Examples of dehumanising, mechanistic and objectifying approaches

In a mixed methods study exploring the impact of the COVID-19 pandemic on ICU staff in Spain, participants reported levels of the "dehumanization of care" (Moreno-Mulet et al., 2021), and whether this is an example of the social system's defences against anxiety or as discussed by Delany and McDougall (2023) is because of moral injury, the results are the same.

In the most extreme situations these defensive behaviours become normalised and institutionalised, and as we have seen repeatedly over time, large-scale cultural collapse can ensue. The many reports of care scandals over the years inevitably describe dehumanisation, objectification and harm to those who use services, their families and the staff involved (Willis, 2020). In 2013, Sir Robert Francis, who led the Public Inquiry into the care failings at Mid Staffordshire NHS Foundation Trust, highlighted the dangers of losing sight of human concerns in healthcare (Francis, 2013). In his landmark report, he emphasised the importance of listening to patients and staff, and the risks to patients when the delivery of care becomes highly depersonalised. During the Inquiry, one junior doctor – now a consultant – told the hearing that the A&E department at Stafford Hospital had become "immune to the sound of pain" (Lintern, 2023).

Dame Elizabeth Buggins in her evidence to the Francis Inquiry commented:

In healthcare organisations, calm confidence is prized and the system has honed its ability to achieve it. Emerging issues, which exacerbate anxiety – like safety concerns, near misses and actual errors – are therefore often not welcome.

In this context there is a risk that people are too keen to be easily reassured and therefore close down difficult conversations and questions too early. This frustrates those who have concerns and speak up, while others become accustomed to deficiencies and dangerously accepting and passive.

Many believe that the hard truths learned through the Francis Inquiry are in danger of being forgotten in the light of unprecedented, continuing and seemingly endless service pressures. The ambient anxiety that is created as a result – unless mitigated – will inevitably have a rapid and negative effect on quality. A decade on from the publication of his report Francis continues to express concerns about a culture of fear and persecution at the highest level of the NHS, with an over-emphasis on top-down command and control approaches to management. He has also expressed significant concern about the lack of basic attention to staff wellbeing, commenting: "The pressure on the human beings who provide the service is such, from top to bottom in any given organisation, that inhumane things are bound to start happening and are happening on a much wider scale than we had at Mid Staffs" (Lintern, 2023). Others argue that some evidence exists for aggregate improvement across the healthcare system since Mid Staffs, citing a number of policy initiatives that were launched in the wake of the Public Inquiry. However they remain uncertain as to whether these were driven by the policy response (Martin et al., 2023).

Francis emphasised the urgency of transforming the culture of NHS organisations away from one that is fearful and defensive and towards one that is open, honest and willing to listen. But perhaps this exhortation for cultural change misses the fundamental point of Menzies-Lyth's work. That is to say that she saw these issues not as individual moral or cultural failures, but as entirely understandable structural defences of the system, built up to protect staff against the worst effects of their emotional labour in specific contexts. Although Menzies-Lyth conducted her research in 1960, her observations feel as relevant today as when they were first published.

Unconscious Processes and the Primary Task of Caring Organisations

Drawing on similar psychoanalytical thinking as Menzies-Lyth, Lawrence (1977) postulated that the primary task that people perform in institutions can be distinguished in three ways. First is the normative task, which is what the institution is explicitly designed to do at a conscious level. Second is the existential task, which is what employees think they do and how they interpret the work and give meaning to their roles and activities. And finally, the phenomenological or the observed task, which relates to what – through observation – they can be said to be doing. Skowrońska (2023) reminds us that when considering the primary task of caring institutions, we must also consider the way that societies unconsciously assign them special functions, which are often associated with the containment of universal human fears. By assigning specific roles to these institutions, she argues that we exempt ourselves from having to deal with difficult issues. As we have already discussed, healthcare environments can become saturated by exhausting and unbearable emotional experiences, and some would argue that the healthcare system serves as a socially sanctioned form of the collective denial of death, with an unspoken promise to treat and extend life no matter what. The phrase "we'll do everything we can" is a well-rehearsed part of the script, which probably means quite different things to professionals than to patients or their families, and yet the meaning is largely unexplored.

Within the group analytical tradition (Foulkes, 2018) the notion of the matrix or the social unconscious (Hopper, 2003; Roberts, 1982) is used to describe the place where we store such connections; a "pattern of intersubjective narrative themes that organise and are organised by the experience of being together, formed through repetitive patterns of communicative action between human bodies" (Stacey, 2003, p. 238). Through healthy projection and mirroring mechanisms – the processes through which a person sees themselves, or part of themselves literally reflected in the interactions of other group members – people share their anxieties, making them easier to bear (Anderson-Wallace, 2017). Creating the spaces and relationships to enable this to happen safely becomes especially important. Furthermore, a clear awareness of the burden created by the inevitable suffering of these environments is crucial. Obholzer and Roberts (1994) describe the need to create the proper conditions for the "psychological dust" generated to be metabolised, rather than simply inhaled. In addition, they remark that clarity about the organisation's task and authority structure, with clear opportunities for the teams to take part in the decision-making process, is also important when working in psychologically demanding settings.

Personal Defences and Wounded Healers

Skowrońska (2023), continuing in the group analytical tradition, argues that an added source of difficulty stems from the fact that it is not uncommon for people who engage in caring work to choose the work as a way of working on their own unresolved problems. She argues that the emotional impact of their work can trigger their specific personal defence mechanisms, which affect functioning not only in relation to patients but also within the teams that they work. As a result of the impact of unrecognised projective processes – the mechanism by which we displace our own feelings and locate them in others – teams can become "caught" in these dynamics without being aware of it. Furthermore, people who choose a helping profession often have experienced relational trauma in their development, especially role reversal. Thus, they develop a kind of "helping self" which enables them to cope by helping others rather than paying attention to their own needs. This can mean that they are paradoxically less likely to seek help to process difficult feelings and responses, and then if these important stories of identity become compromised by their inability to cope, the results can be catastrophic. Nitsun (2001) describes something similar in considering the wounded healer phenomenon, developing an archetype first developed by Swiss psychiatrist Carl Jung. He notes that wounded healers are often intuitive and insightful but can also be vulnerable. Their suffering often starts with overwork and the exhaustion it causes. This, in turn, results in feelings of helplessness and frustration, followed by guilt, and feelings that they have failed in their caring role. They can also feel trapped by the complex and sometimes contradictory needs of their patients (Nitsun, 2001), and grasping this complexity is difficult and takes time – time that is often not available in busy caring environments (Skowrońska, 2023). As the goal of caring well for people becomes unreachable, the risk of people retreating into professional personas and becoming emotionally distanced is heightened. As important elements of personal identity – their aspirations, hopes and dreams for their caring work – are denied and repressed, work becomes devoid of meaning. If not recognised the level of mental distress can become unbearable. According to Viktor Frankl, a psychiatrist who managed to survive the Nazi concentration camps, there is no reason for healthcare professionals to be ashamed of their suffering. Skowrońska (2023, p.10) citing Frankl argues that "just like destiny or death, suffering is a fundamental human experience. If life has meaning, then suffering must necessarily have meaning too". According to Frankl, when a person accepts their destiny and suffering, this can provide life with a profound sense of meaning (Frankl, 1985).

If we accept the immense psychological and emotional risk that is associated with caring work, and we accept that suffering is a central dimension of the caring role, then it follows that we must develop the organisational frameworks, routines and practices to support this. The institutionalisation of practices that lessen the pervasive anxiety of caring work, ending the need for these structural defences, should therefore be a priority to ensure quality.

Balint Groups, Reflective Practice and Schwartz Rounds

Practices that aim to tackle the emotional and psychological challenges of healthcare work have been present in the NHS for a long time. Balint groups – named after the psychoanalyst Michael Balint – originated in the 1950s when groups of family doctors met on a regular basis with a trained facilitator to discuss any subject that came to mind outside of their typical clinical encounters (Balint, 1955). These groups could have several aims, but the central belief was that by having a better understanding of how they were affected by the emotional content of caring for patients, doctors would be better able to actively process – and thus successfully provide – relationship-centred care. Numerous studies have shown that taking part in a Balint group can improve the participant's capacity for coping, psychological awareness and patient centredness (Kjeldmand & Holmström, 2008; Kjeldmand et al., 2004). In mental health settings long-term staff support groups are common and it is argued that such work done diligently over time gradually changes the team culture (Skowrońska, 2023). That said these groups take time to mature, but if the teams can safely explore the various levels of the group matrix (Foulkes, 2018) and make healthy connections between them, then it is possible not just to contain difficult feelings arising from the work, but also to enrich the professional work of team members.

Schwartz Rounds are organisation-wide forums that prompt reflection and discussion of the emotional, social and ethical challenges of healthcare work, with the aim of improving staff wellbeing and patient care. They were introduced into the UK in 2009 to support healthcare staff to deliver compassionate care.

According to the Point of Care Foundation (n.d.), that led the UK development and spread of the approach, the purpose of "Rounds" is to understand the challenges and rewards that are intrinsic to providing care, not to solve problems or to focus on the clinical aspects of patient care. They claim that Rounds can help staff feel more supported in their jobs, allowing them the time and space to reflect on their roles. Evidence shows that staff who attend Rounds feel less stressed and isolated, with increased insight and appreciation for each other's roles. They also help to reduce hierarchies between staff and to focus attention on relational aspects of care. The underlying premise for Rounds is that the compassion shown by staff can make all the difference to a patient's experience of care, but that in order to provide compassionate care staff must, in turn, feel supported in their work. The network expanded in the aftermath of the Francis Inquiry, and Rounds are now run in hundreds of healthcare organisations all over the NHS. Evidence is emerging that this approach, which encourages an explicit focus on the emotional toll of caring work, is valuable.

Each Round has a topic or patient focus and a title that is shared in advance in publicity material, and lasts for one hour, is preceded by food and begins with a multi-disciplinary panel presentation. Each panel member focuses on their own experiences in relation to the emotional and psychological impact of caring for patients and their families and any issues arising in terms of working with colleagues. Together with a clinical lead, a trained facilitator guides the discussion of emerging themes and issues, allowing time and space for the audience and panel to reflect and talk about similar experiences that they have had. Attendance is voluntary, open to all and staff attend as many or as few Rounds as they would like, with attendance varying from 10 to over 100.

Robert et al. (2017) conclude that Rounds were typically adopted to improve staff wellbeing and that adopting organisations scored better on staff engagement than non-adopters. Among adopting organisations, those performing better on existing patient experience measures were more likely to adopt earlier. A generally favourable set of innovation attributes (including low cost), advocacy from opinion leaders in different professional networks, active dissemination by change agents and a felt need to be seen to be addressing staff wellbeing led to Rounds being seen as "an idea whose time had come". More recent adoption patterns have been shaped by the timing of charitable and other agency funding in specific geographical areas and sectors, as well as several forms of "mimetic pressure" – the processes that encourage imitation within and between organisations and encourage staff through peer processes to conform. A realist-informed mixed methods evaluation of Schwartz Rounds in England concluded that healthcare staff who regularly attended Rounds to share the emotional, social, or ethical challenges they face in the workplace experience less psychological distress, improved teamwork and increased empathy and compassion for patients and colleagues (Maben et al., 2018). A subsequent study quantified this, suggesting that attendance was linked to a 19% reduction in psychological distress adjusting for covariates. Dawson et al. (2021) concluded that as an organisation-wide intervention, Rounds constituted an effective, relatively low-cost intervention to assist staff in dealing with the demands of their work and to improve their wellbeing (Dawson et al., 2021).

Moral Distress and Injury

If we accept that the quality of the care is highly dependent on the members of staff being psychologically and emotionally, as well as physically, present, then it follows that if they are put under very sustained pressure, they may feel unable to offer the care they believe is needed. This predicament has been described as a position of "moral distress", where the tension of not being able to act in ways that feel morally right becomes overwhelming. Research has shown that in these situations staff sensitivity to stress and burnout is significantly heightened (Morley et al., 2019). This has obvious implications and ultimately risks creating a situation where it becomes incrementally harder to provide high-quality care as precious capacity is continually reduced by sickness, absence, recruitment and retention, leading in turn to further pressure on those "still standing".

Much of the literature regarding moral injury has arisen from the trauma experienced by those working in conflict zones. Specifically cited is the clinical research relating to existential crises experienced by war veterans. This work describes the "character wounds" that annihilate trust and have a detrimental effect on a person's moral foundations (Shay, 2003, 2010). The clinical presentation is thought to be distinct from post-traumatic stress disorder and to be more intricately linked to the systemic effects of managerial and executive decisions, where there is a sense of betrayal that someone in a position of legitimate authority has not acted to safeguard the conditions necessary for safe, effective and individualised care (Shay, 2014). This can also involve intentionally making choices that place practitioners in the role of perpetrators; those who fail to stop acts, as well as bearing witness to or learning about activities that go against their sincerely held moral standards and expectations (Litz et al., 2009). This clash of moral worlds can be readily seen within public services and has become the focus of increased study and reflection during and after the COVID-19 pandemic (Shale, 2020). Shale emphasises that moral injury can be experienced by anybody – including patients and family members – by introducing a larger concept of moral injury based on moral philosophy. According to this definition, moral harm results from a variety of causes, such as injustice, cruelty, status degradation, and a grave violation of accepted moral standards. Shale describes how our everyday moral life is shaped by normative expectations, or our views about what "should" happen paired with predictions about what "will" happen. She contends that when these expectations are realised, people can have faith, hope and confidence in the future, and when they are not, the risk of moral harm is increased and confusion, embarrassment and resentment are all too easy to feel (Shale, 2020). There is an obvious link here to harm in the healthcare context as it is fundamentally linked to breaches in normative expectations (Anderson-Wallace & Shale, 2014a). Citing Greenberg and Tracy, Shale (2020) points out that preventive psychological approaches to supporting staff in healthcare environments can help to mitigate the risk of occupational moral injury. This entails strengthening relationships between co-workers and supervisors, successfully providing for the basic requirements of the workforce, and being alert to the first indications of distress. Also, they stress the significance of viewing responses as genuine and meaningful rather than "medicalising" or pathologising them.

Importantly, psychological debriefing methods – particularly those which are reactive and one-off – have been found to be ineffective, and in some cases actively harmful (Rose et al., 2003). It is therefore important to give attention to how these types of interventions can be institutionalised; where responsibility is taken at an organisational and not merely individual level; and where the remedies are built into the everyday workflow.

Shale proposes an approach to moral repair which can be preventive as well as reparative and aims to re-establish a sense of moral equilibrium within individuals and between people (Greenberg & Tracy, 2020, cited in Shale, 2020). Two specific leadership proprieties are identified as central to this process. The first is the inquisitorial, which promotes a fair and impartial process of investigation which "enables an objective record of the morally relevant facts" (Shale, 2011, p. 141) to be established. The second is the restorative, which focuses on the processes that help return moral relationships to balance. This involves bearing witness to the narratives of wrong; accepting grief and anger as a normal part of the process of healing, and clear notions of categorical apology (Smith, 2008) and forgiveness (Cantacuzino, 2015). Delany and McDougall (2023) discuss this further, citing the developing evidence that facilitated ethics discussions in groups can increase the sense of moral agency and professional integrity. They further argue that building a sense of a moral community can help professionals to develop a stronger collective voice, enabling greater advocacy for organisational and policy changes. It is interesting to note the emphasis that is placed on the need to develop a strong sense of genuine curiosity in this work; a theme that we strongly advocate throughout this book.

Defensive Practice

In a context of rising demand and shrinking resources, it is easy to see how a complex mix of ambient pressures can push clinicians, managers and other staff to behave defensively, and in ways which to the lay person seem antithetical to the delivery of compassionate, patient-centred care. Much has been written about the effects of the perceived increases in litigation and complaints in the healthcare context and the defensive response from practitioners (Ortashi et al., 2013; Studdert et al., 2005; Toker et al., 2004). Accounts of ambulance-chasing lawyers and demanding or entitled patients who are unable or unwilling to accept the limitations of services or their own conditions all feed into a narrative that can drive defensive practice.

The definition of defensive medicine is when a doctor departs from accepted practice to lessen or avoid complaints or criticism (Toker et al., 2004). Clinical experts claim that this results in unnecessary referrals and deferrals, excess diagnostic testing, and overtreatment. According to studies, 78% to 93% of doctors practise defensive medicine, so the potential cost associated with this is not difficult to imagine – pure Failure Demand. According to Berwick and Hackbarth (2012) around a third of medicine is waste, with no measurable effects or justification for the considerable expenditure incurred. This is a stark figure when considered carefully. The crucial point here is whether this defensive positioning exposes patients to added risk from the unnecessary and often invasive treatments, risks which may be higher than that of missing an unlikely diagnosis.

Thorpe (2004) argues that paternalism and self-regulation have long been a part of medicine and as citizens become more self-assured and informed about their options, some doctors, who are unaccustomed to having their ethical standards and professional judgement questioned, have experienced significant difficulties adjusting to this. Ortashi et al. (2013) argue that citizens have also grown more risk-averse while becoming better informed, often refusing to acknowledge the generally low likelihood of unfavourable outcomes associated with medical treatment and interventions. Brilla et al. (2006) claim that this encourages medical personnel to avoid potentially dangerous activities, prompting them to adopt a defensive position and request tests not for medical reasons but rather to lessen the possibility of complaints or legal action. If there is litigation, a "more defendable" case is produced, at the very least (Brilla et al., 2006). According to Chen (2007), this tactic is complicated by the assumption that courts often depend on investigational evidence rather than declarations of experience or medical judgement (Chen, 2007). Moreover, negative defensive medicine (such as limiting or denying care or treatment to patients deemed too "risky" by physicians) may be a factor in health system inequality.

There is no doubt that clinicians hold one another and themselves to exacting standards. Despite the clear prevalence of human error, no one likes the idea that they have made a mistake, and the stakes are higher when someone may be hurt as a result – possibly gravely or fatally. But there is also a clear undercurrent in professional cultures that is founded on the idea of infallibility and characterised by intolerance for any departure from it (Goldman, 2010). One of the main reasons offered for not reporting clinical incidents is the fear of being personally blamed (Vincent et al., 1999). Despite being rare, recent prosecutions for gross negligence manslaughter have led to an elevated sense of fear and anxiety, producing tremendous disquiet throughout the healthcare professions (Williams, 2018). According to Lucian Leape, the so-called father of patient safety, the single biggest obstacle to improvements in patient safety is the effects of medical culture.

The Fear of Litigation

At present medical injury claims in the UK can be made through tort litigation, with payments obtained by court orders or out-of-court agreements. When clinicians receive a complaint or are involved in litigation, the reaction is often intensely personal. Affected clinicians may experience feelings of rage, remorse, embarrassment and loss of confidence, and some even consider leaving the profession (Robertson & Thomson, 2014). The negative effects on claimants' physical and mental health, as well as their incomes, are also well documented (Delbanco & Bell 2007; Vandersteegen et al., 2015).

The NHS in England spends more than £2 billion annually on paying people who were harmed during treatment, and the system costs have been increasing at an alarming rate. Ten years ago, the NHS paid damages totalling £900 million; in 2022, it was £2.17 billion, which is equal to the annual operating expenses of the largest hospital trust in England. During the next ten years, this amount is expected to quadruple with legal fees accounting for about a quarter of these expenses. Clinical negligence costs the English NHS 2% of its overall revenue (Health and Social Care Committee, 2022). The same Select Committee Inquiry concluded that processes that are supposed to deliver justice and incentivise improvements fail to do either, with lessons rarely being learned, and for families accessing compensation the experience was slow, adversarial, stressful and often bitter. Furthermore, they claim that the outcomes are often arbitrary – based not on need but on whether clinical negligence can be proved.

To counter the negative effects of litigation and to limit the costs to the public purse, several countries – most notably in the Nordic countries and New Zealand – have introduced no fault compensation schemes (NFCS) that enable harmed patients to be compensated without the need to prove negligence. These schemes and the motivation for having them are complex but importantly include:

- The more precise targeting of compensation for intended beneficiaries (Davis et al., 2002)
- The impacts on physical and mental health outcomes (Cameron et al., 2008) and health system costs (Dickson, 2016)
- The more equitable access to justice (Bismark et al., 2006a, 2006b) and healthcare (Dubay et al., 1999)
- The importance of procedural justice (Siegal et al., 2008)
- The possibilities of improved patient safety (Wallis, 2013)

Measuring the effectiveness of schemes to meet all these aims is, however, extremely complex. A recent review of litigation reform proved that the effects of these schemes remain highly contested (Health and Social Care Committee, 2022).

The Review's main proposal was for the NHS to implement a fundamentally different system for compensating harmed patients, one that shifts away from a system centred on assigning blame towards one which places a higher priority on learning from mistakes.

In the most serious circumstances, they propose that a separate administrative authority – not the courts – should oversee conducting investigations and deciding who qualifies for compensation. The Bar Council for England said that to suggest that clinical negligence should generate learning "is to misunderstand the purpose of tort law (addressing wrongs) which is to compensate the victim and not to punish or prevent recidivism by the Tortfeasor" (Health and Social Care Committee, 2022, p. 20), and that to introduce a new statutory administrative scheme would be "a project of phenomenal ambition" (Health and Social Care Committee, 2022, p. 24).

Safety and Healthcare Harm

Since the Institute of Medicine (IoM) report "To Err is Human" (Donaldson et al., 2000) the issue of system safety and reducing healthcare harm has been in focus for health systems all over the world. In the NHS, the IoM report was mirrored by the landmark report from the Chief Medical Officer (Donaldson, 2002; Eva & Regher, 2000) which looked at what was known about the scope and character of healthcare harm in the UK, as well as what might be learnt from past mistakes. Both reports introduced notions of clinical error for the first time and placed an emphasis on unified reporting channels, a more open culture and ensuring that lessons learned were incorporated. A systems-based approach to reducing error was proposed, drawing on knowledge and experience from other high-risk industries, but in practice many argue that the focus on clinical error achieved the exact opposite (Wears & Sutcliffe, 2019).

In the NHS in England, the National Patient Safety Agency was set up, whose role was to implement the findings of the report and ensure that lessons were learnt and fed back into practice. A cornerstone of the new approach to patient safety was a system of reporting, recording, analysing and learning from error. Over the next 20 years, significant efforts were made to develop such systems all over the world, and yet despite all the activity, investment and improvement effort, rates of healthcare harm appear to have remained stable and progress in reducing harm has been glacially slow (Illingworth et al., 2022; Wears & Sutcliffe, 2019).

Hollnagel et al. (2015) argue that this can be attributed to the way in which safety itself has been defined; making a distinction between what they call Safety I and Safety II, which can be summarised as shown in Table 10.1.

They argue that there is an urgent need to modify our approach to safety considering the rising demands and expanding system complexity. While a Safety I failure can still be used to understand many adverse events, this perspective neglects to consider the fact that human performance almost always goes according to plan. Things go well not because people act appropriately (i.e. correctly follow the rules or processes), but rather because they modify their behaviour to suit the circumstances of their particular work scenario. These modifications become more crucial to maintain acceptable performance as systems become more interdependent and complex. Understanding how adaptations are made, or how performance typically goes well despite the uncertainties, ambiguities, and goal conflicts that permeate complicated work circumstances, is the challenge for safety improvement.

Whilst the distinction between Safety I and Safety II is now common in the literature, much of the organisational and institutional practice is still predicated on the former, despite the conditions suggesting the latter may be more beneficial and effective. Wears and Sutcliffe (2019) argue that the reason for this is that the patient safety movement in healthcare remains dominated by the disciplines of medicine and management and has failed to properly integrate and use the knowledge of other domains, which have been highly influential in safety science in other industries – especially psychology, sociology and engineering.

Table 10.1 Safety I and Safety II (adapted from Finkel, 2011; Hollnagel et al., 2015)

	Safety I	Safety II
Central beliefs about causation	Things go wrong because of identifiable failures or malfunctions of specific components, be they technology, procedures, the human workers or the organisations in which they are embedded	Things go right most of the time due to system flexibility and resilience. Complexity and interdependence mean effects can be described but linear causation is impossible to establish
Approach	Ways of working that minimise the likelihood of accidents and incidents and reducing the level of risk to an acceptable level	Ways of working that enhance the system ability to succeed under varying conditions. Building resilience into system design enables safety to become a system property
Focus	Focus efforts into methods that ensure that 'as few things as possible go wrong'	Focus on method that ensures that 'as many things as possible go right'
	Manage people and conditions to prevent them making mistakes in the future	To facilitate everyday work, anticipate developments and events, and to maintain the adaptive capacity to respond effectively to inevitable surprises
	Respond when something happens or is categorised as an unacceptable risk, usually by trying to eliminate causes or improve barriers, or both	
View of humans	Humans are the most unpredictable variable, and whether acting alone or in groups are therefore primarily seen as a liability or hazard. Humans are the "weak" points in the system	Humans are basically good at making the everyday performance adaptations that are needed to respond to varying conditions - this is why things go mostly right. Humans are the "glue" that makes things work
Tools and techniques	Risk assessment aims to predict problems and control variation ahead of things going wrong. Identification of violations in standard operating procedures allows for corrections to be made	Dynamic risk assessment to understand conditions where performance variability becomes difficult or impossible to control. Identifying patterns that are resilient and flexible and amplifying them
Approach to investigation	Discover the root causes and contributing elements of undesirable outcomes. Make specific recommendations to resolve them	Learning to develop an understanding of how things usually go right, since that is the basis for explaining how things occasionally go wrong

Compounded Harm

There is little doubt that we have some significant problems when it comes to providing consistently safe and reliable care. When things go wrong our current models often inadvertently make the restoration of trust and the repair of the relationship both more difficult and costly in both financial and human terms.

Numerous patient safety inquiry reports over recent years have consistently provided powerful evidence that people who have already suffered the most devastating consequences of unsafe healthcare are also routinely caused further harm by the way the system responds (Francis, 2013; Kirkup, 2015; Vize, 2022). In a recent survey conducted by the Harmed Patient Alliance over 80% either "disagreed" or "strongly disagreed" that they had been "seen and heard as if they truly mattered since the harm happened". Not a single respondent felt that they were treated with the care, compassion, kindness and respect they had expected from the NHS. Many described being forced to fight for answers, with prolonged and profound impacts including serious mistrust in their ongoing relationship with healthcare; 86% reported impacts on working life, 83% on physical health and 69% on personal relationships. More than 90% of respondents said that the organisation's response negatively impacted on their mental health and/or emotional and psychological wellbeing, and 94% stated that they had to find and/or pay for emotional, practical or psychological support to help try to recover from what happened to them – harm that was created by the service that was there to heal them. In summary, the responses indicate that for most, the organisation's actions caused "compounded harm" with significant negative impacts on healing, wellbeing, trust and relationships (Titcombe et al., 2023). They argue that dealing with "harmed" patients and their families appears in some way exempt from the obligations expressed in the NHS values, evidenced by a lack of systemic action to avoid compounded harm. Whilst being honest when things go wrong and showing compassion when participating in learning or investigative processes are crucial, minimising "compounded harm" is about much more than that. The report calls for a more fundamental rethinking of what is required to "heal" (to restore wellness, trust and just relationships following healthcare injury); as well as for organisations to assume proper responsibility for their actions in the interests of justice (Hughes et al., 2023). Although "restorative just culture" has featured more prominently in the patient safety discourse of late, this has been seen largely as an antidote to the "blame game" that is believed to suppress staff openness and therefore impact on organisational learning (Cribb et al., 2022). Recent literature is largely silent on the issue of attending to the healing needs of patients and their families, remaining focused on primacy of organisational learning or staff wellbeing (Dekker et al., 2022). If we consider the aftermath of harm as being about staff and harmed patients and family wellbeing, as well as organisational learning, then a "just" response they argue must include a complex process of moral repair that is an expression of the espoused values of the NHS (Hughes et al., 2023).

Restorative Approaches

The restorative approach is based on the philosophy that justice is created not by punishing those who broke the rules but by repairing the harm caused. It recognises that clinical staff are often very deeply affected by events, and strategies aimed at ensuring their wellbeing, trust and relationships with their employer, colleagues and role after things have gone wrong are critical. It therefore follows that harmed patients and families also deserve a "restorative and just" response to their wellbeing, trust and relationship needs too, and a failure to do this will further compound harm and generate an even greater sense of injustice. It is tempting to think that we can plan, train, measure and/or regulate ourselves out of this situation, and whilst these elements may have a part to play, a more fundamental disruption of the prevailing institutional attitudes and beliefs is needed, including significant investment in infrastructure. This is a challenging "ask" in the current circumstances, but the human and moral arguments are compelling, and the financial costs to the system undeniable. A much deeper conversation about healing – the restoration of wellbeing, trust and just relationships with all those affected after healthcare harm – is needed. This is likely to be a difficult conversation, which touches on many "taboos" and challenges to the existing public discourse around safety in healthcare. It is a conversation that will need the commitment of many across the public, political, clinical and regulatory space.

Promoting Organisational Effectiveness

Many argue that building organisational health and developing restorative just cultures are crucial to this argument (Dekker et al., 2022). These approaches focus on the creation of psychological safety in the workplace conditions, enabling interpersonal risk in relationships, and encouraging ethical frameworks for practice, including the freedom to name issues before they become a considerable risk (Edmondson, 2018; Martin et al., 2021). There is no doubt that proactively supporting those who raise concerns is also considered to be important and this type of prosocial organisational behaviour (Miceli et al., 2008; Shale & Anderson-Wallace, 2020) can also help to create the conditions for a shift away from "comfort seeking" approaches to risk, towards more pro-active "problem sensing" methods (Cullen, 2016; Dixon-Woods et al., 2014). However, there is a broader context and all of this must be supported by an intelligent, fair and compassionate approach to professional regulation, and a just approach to support and investigation when things go wrong (Wailling et al., 2022). Dekker et al. (2022) consider the experience of Mersey Care, a large provider of Mental Health and Community Care support in the Northwest of England, as an exemplar of an organisation that has used the aim of building a restorative just culture to build organisational resilience. There is little doubt that the work has been impressive with tangible outcomes in terms of practical and economic benefits (Kaur et al., 2019), however despite significant publicity the models used do not appear to have become widespread.

Anderson-Wallace and Shale (2014a) conducted an analysis of the Francis Public Inquiry report and found 50 recommendations that refer to work that care organisations should be doing on a continuing basis to help rebuild trust following perceived failures in the care they provide. They suggest seven ethical practices that organisations should focus on when aiming to build an environment of quality in response to healthcare harm. At the heart of these practices is a research-based understanding of the moral relationship that exists between patients and healthcare organisations. The ethical practices provide an integrated account of the steps that it is necessary to take to build and, when necessary, rebuild, confidence, trust and hope, and promote a proactive approach to making amends and supporting professional staff, so that the consequences of healthcare harm are less devastating for everyone involved. Each practice has a detailed descriptor that addresses all three dimensions of quality – effectiveness, safety and experience – by asking core questions as outlined in Figure 10.3.

Effectiveness:	Safety:	Experience:
Why are we doing this, and therefore what should our actions focus on?	What do we need to do to ensure safe care for this and other patients?	How do we want people affected to experience our actions?

1	Attentiveness to negative perceptions of care, and supportive action in response to complaints
2	Supportive disclosure to patients and their supporters
3	Support for clinicians, clinical teams and other affected staff
4	Transparent, impartial and authoritative enquiry
5	Implementation of actions approved and collaboratively developed with patients and supporters
6	Restorative approach to restitution
7	Institutional and individual accountability

Figure 10.3   Seven ethical practices (Anderson-Wallace & Shale, 2014b)

Many of Francis' proposals were put into practice as part of the policy response. The need that providers select a "freedom to speak up" guardian to promote openness and guarantee people's complaints are heard, and the legislative responsibility of candour on the part of provider organisations when patients are harmed, were both swiftly adopted. The method of inspection used by the Care Quality Commission was changed. Frameworks for responding to patient safety incidents also underwent two significant changes. But many of the recommendations did not result in changes to policy. For instance, guidelines on minimum staffing ratios have still not been implemented despite mounting evidence (Griffiths & Dall'Ora, 2022) and long-term financial and workforce issues, combined with post-pandemic strains on services, have made safe staffing increasingly politically problematic. As Martin et al. (2023) note, evaluations of the changes made are uncommon, and when they have been done (for instance, on openness initiatives in trusts) organisational commitment and capability have varied. More than ten years on from the publication of the Francis Public Inquiry report, implementation of the 50 recommendations that Anderson-Wallace & Shale refer to in their ethical practices framework has been extremely limited.

Blame, Shame and Justice

The culture of "blame" and "shame" that persists discourages openness and learning (Waring, 2005) and although there is a growing awareness of the needs of both families and of professionals involved in harm events, the practical infrastructure to support alternative ways of working are generally not available. Of course, the situation is complex as there are many audiences – coroners, commissioners, professional and system regulators – who may not share the same interests and/or have statutory roles to play which conflict with others. As Cribb et al. (2022) note, organisations may officially support "no blame" rhetoric but in day-to-day operations personnel may still feel they are being treated unfairly. They might also formally admit that the system caused the injury, but a family might view this as a way of individuals being held accountable and as an avoidance of proper sanctions. Families and professionals may also be concerned about the efficacy or value of some types of "moral repair" when there does not appear to be a sincere admission of fault on anyone's behalf. Cribb et al. (2022) argue that we need to make many of these debates more concrete and advocate "real world" policies and practices that ask what ideas about justice (in which combinations) they embody. This conversation could explore proportionate sanctions, shared learning and accountability, and repairing damage, as well as asking about the relative importance of these different values and how best to balance and combine them in practice. In conclusion, they suggest that everyone involved in enhancing the safety of healthcare should carefully and openly consider the ethical balancing acts requiring interpretations of justice through retributive (with sanctions), distributive (no blame or qualified blame) and reparative (focused on healing) lenses.

Aubin and King (2018) consider healthcare as an ecosystem that is perfect for growing shame. They define shame as a complex array of cognitive, perceptual and emotional phenomena, as an "assault of the self" (Van Vliet, 2008, p. 237), and "one of the most powerful, painful and potentially destructive experiences known to humans" (Gilbert, 1997, p. 113). Shame is the result of comparing oneself to an internal standard or ideal; it follows that the higher the standards one has, the more likely a person will encounter the feeling of shame. As previously discussed, healthcare professionals have exceptionally exacting standards overall, and coupled with the "yoke of perfection" (Hilfiker, 1984) and a general lack of acceptance of fallibility, the conditions for shame to thrive are obvious. The dynamic of both internal erosion of identity and the external exposure associated with admissions of error has an unmasking effect. But shame can also be a force which enables reassessment and a reconnection with one's own sense of human-ity, assuming that it is handled in the right way by colleagues and collaborators. Aubin and King (2018) argue that what is required is not a "just culture", but an empathetic one, as empathy can help to reshape the mask of infallibility and act as a reminder that healthcare professionals are not alone in their struggle in a complex, unpredictable and demanding profession.

Conclusion

In this chapter we have considered a wide range of issues that create the context for unhelpful patterns of behaviour that significantly affect relationships, adversely influence the context of care and create defensive practice, and have reflected on a range of evidence-based approaches which can make a considerable difference. We have spent a good deal of time considering healthcare harm, which is one of the biggest areas of Failure Demand in the healthcare system. A great deal of empha-sis is placed on the need for "lessons to be learnt" in relation to this domain, yet all of the formal systems developed to report and learn have failed to deliver the expected results. The tacit transfer of complex knowledge between actors within the work system is crucial to this, and investment in developing social and relational systems is of critical importance. We have argued that the institutionalisation of approaches to ethical, restorative and reflective practices is a prerequisite for this type of learning and is more likely to support sustainable changes. Contemporary notions of professional accountability and a context of greater sharing of respon-sibility, knowledge equity and decision-making amongst all those involved in care – including patients, their families and wider social networks – can help reframe the work and improve quality (Elwyn et al., 2012; Gilbert, 2019). It is clear however that these approaches are in their infancy in most organisations in the NHS.

Acknowledgements

We would like to specifically acknowledge Dr Suzanne Shale, whose scholarship and work with Murray Anderson-Wallace in the wake of the Mid-Staffordshire Public Inquiry shaped much of the thinking that informed this chapter.

References

Anderson-Wallace, M. 2017. *Mirroring in Groupwork Practice*. Occasional Paper. Institute of Group Analysis.

Anderson-Wallace, M. and Shale, S. 2014a. *Draft Ethical Practices for the Management of Perceived, Suspected or Known Medical Errors or Harm*. Occasional Paper. Leeds University.

Anderson-Wallace, M. and Shale, S. 2014b. Restoring trust: What is "quality" in the aftermath of healthcare harm? *Clinical Risk*, 20(1–2): 16–18.

Aubin, D. and King, S. 2018. The healthcare environment: A perfect ecosystem for growing shame. *Healthcare Quarterly*, 20: 31–36.

Balint, M. 1955. The doctor, his patient, and the illness. *The Lancet*, 265(6866): 683–688.

Berwick, D.M. and Hackbarth, A.D. 2012. Eliminating waste in US health care. *JAMA*, 307: 1513–1516. doi: 10.1001/jama.2012.362

Bismark, M.M., Brennan, T.A., Davis, P.B. and Studdert, D.M. 2006a. Claiming behaviour in a no-fault system of medical injury: A descriptive analysis of claimants and nonclaimants. *Medical Journal of Australia*, 185(4): 203–207.

Bismark, M.M., Brennan, T.A., Paterson, R.J., Davis, P.B. and Studdert, D.M. 2006b. Relationship between complaints and quality of care in New Zealand: A descriptive analysis of complaints and non-complaints following adverse events. *Quality and Safety in Health Care*, 15: 17–22.

Brilla, R., Evers, S., Deutschländer, A. and Wartenberg, K.E. 2006. Are neurology residents in the United States being taught defensive medicine. *Clinical Neurology and Neurosurgery*, 108(4): 374–377.

Burgess, N., Currie, G., Crump, B. and Dawson, A. 2022. Leading change across a healthcare system: How to build improvement capability and foster a culture of continuous improvement: Lessons from an evaluation of the NHS-VMI partnership. Warwick Business School.

Cameron, I.D., Rebbeck, T., Sindhusake, D., Rubin, G., Feyer, A., Walsh, J. and Schofield, W.N. 2008. Legislative change is associated with improved health status in people with whiplash. *Spine*, 33: 250–254.

Cantacuzino, M. 2015. *The Forgiveness Project: Stories for a Vengeful Age*. Jessica Kingsley Publishers.

Chambliss, D.F. 1996. *Beyond Caring: Hospitals, Nurses, and the Social Organization of Ethics*. University of Chicago Press.

Chen, X.Y. 2007. Defensive medicine or economically motivated corruption? A Confucian reflection on physician care in China today. *Journal of Medicine and Philosophy*, 32(6): 635–648.

Cornwell, J. 2021. Reflections on 15 years of the Point of Care. https://www.pointofcarefoundation.org.uk/blog/reflections-on-15-years-of-the-point-of-care/

Cribb, A., O'Hara, J.K. and Waring, J. 2022. Improving responses to safety incidents: We need to talk about justice. *BMJ Quality & Safety*, 31(4): 327–330.

Cullen, A. 2016. Schwartz Rounds – Promoting compassionate care and healthy organisations. *Journal of Social Work Practice*, 30(2): 219–228.

Daneault, S. 2008. The wounded healer: Can this idea be of use to family physicians? *Canadian Family Physician*, 54(9): 1218–1219, 1223–1225.

Davis, P., Lay-Yee, R., Fitzjohn, J., Hider, P., Briant, R. and Schug, S. 2002. Compensation for medical injury in New Zealand: Does "no fault" increase the level of claims-making and reduce its social and clinical selectivity? *Journal of Health Politics, Policy and Law*, 27(5): 833–854.

Dawson, J., McCarthy, I., Taylor, C., Hildenbrand, K., Leamy, M., Reynolds, E. and Maben, J. 2021. Effectiveness of a group intervention to reduce the psychological distress of healthcare staff: A pre-post quasi-experimental evaluation. *BMC Health Services Research*, 21(1): 1–9.

Dekker, S., Oates, A. and Rafferty, J. (eds). 2022. *Restorative Just Culture in Practice: Implementation and Evaluation*. CRC Press.

Delany, C. and McDougall, R. 2023. Support for clinicians with moral loss after the pandemic. *BMJ*, 380: e072629. doi: 10.1136/bmj-2022-072629.

Delbanco, T. and Bell, S.K. 2007. Guilty, afraid, and alone – struggling with medical error. *New England Journal of Medicine*, 357(17): 1682–1683.

Dickson, K.E. 2016. *No-fault Compensation Schemes: A Rapid Realist Review*. EPPI-Centre, Social Science Research Unit, Institute of Education, UCL.

Dixon-Woods, M., Baker, R., Charles, K., Dawson, J., Jerzembek, G., Martin, G., McCarthy, I., McKee, L., Minion, J., Ozieranski, P. and Willars, J. 2014. Culture and behaviour in the English National Health Service: Overview of lessons from a large multimethod study. *BMJ Quality & Safety*, 23(2): 106–115.

Donaldson, L. 2002. An organisation with a memory. *Clinical Medicine*, 2(5): 452.

Donaldson, M.S., Corrigan, J.M. and Kohn, L.T. (eds). 2000. *To Err is Human: Building a Safer Health System*. Institute of Medicine, Committee on Quality of Health Care in America. National Academies Press.

Dubay, L., Kaestner, R. and Waidmann, T. (1999) The impact of malpractice fears on cesarean section rates. *Journal of Health Economics*, 18: 491–522.

Edmondson, A.C. 2018. *The Fearless Organization: Creating Psychological Safety in the Workplace for Learning, Innovation, and Growth*. John Wiley & Sons.

Elwyn, G., Frosch, D., Thomson, R., Joseph-Williams, N., Lloyd, A., Kinnersley, P., Cording, E., Tomson, D., Dodd, C., Rollnick, S. and Edwards, A. 2012. Shared decision making: A model for clinical practice. *Journal of General Internal Medicine*, 27(10): 1361–1367.

Eva, K.W. and Regher, G. 2000. *An Organisation with a Memory: Report of an Expert Group on Learning from Adverse Events in the NHS*. The Stationery Office.

Finkel, M. 2011. *On Flexibility: Recovery from Technological and Doctrinal Surprise on the Battlefield*. Stanford, CA: Stanford University Press.

Foulkes, S.H. 2018. *Therapeutic Group Analysis*. Routledge.

Francis, R. 2013. *Report of the Mid Staffordshire NHS Foundation Trust Public Inquiry: Executive Summary* (Vol. 947). The Stationery Office.

Frankl, V.E. 1985. *Man's Search for Meaning*. Simon and Schuster.

Gilbert, D. 2019. *The Patient Revolution: How We Can Heal the Healthcare System*. Jessica Kingsley Publishers.

Gilbert, P. 1997. The evolution of social attractiveness and its role in shame, humiliation, guilt and therapy. *British Journal of Medical Psychology*, 70: 113–147. doi: 10.1111/j.2044-8341.1997.tb01893.x

Goldman, B. 2010. *Doctors Make Mistakes*. TEDxToronto. www.ted.com/talks/brian_goldman_doctors_make_mistakes_can_we_talk_about_that/transcript?language¼en

Greenberg, N. and Tracy, D. 2020. What healthcare leaders need to do to protect the psychological well-being of frontline staff in the COVID-19 pandemic. *BMJ Leader*. doi: 10.1136/leader-2020-000273

Griffiths, P. and Dall'Ora, C. 2022. Nurse staffing and patient safety in acute hospitals: Cassandra calls again? *BMJ Quality & Safety*. doi: 10.1136/bmjqs-2022-015578

Health and Social Care Committee. 2022. *NHS Litigation Reform*. Thirteenth Report of Session 2021–22. Health and Social Care Committee.

Hilfiker, D. 1984. Facing our mistakes. *New England Journal of Medicine*, 310(2): 118–122. doi: 10.1056/NEJM198401123100211

Hollnagel, E., Wears, R.L. and Braithwaite, J. 2015. *From Safety I to Safety II: A White Paper*. The Resilient Health Care Net – University of Southern Denmark, University of Florida, USA, and Macquarie University, Australia.

Hopper, E. 2003. *The Social Unconscious: Selected Papers* (Vol. 22). Jessica Kingsley Publishers.

Hughes, J., Anderson-Wallace, M. and Titcombe, J. 2023 *Healing After Healthcare Harm: A Call for Restorative Action*. https://harmedpatientsalliance.org.uk/healing-after-healthcare-harm-a-call-for-restorative-action/

Illingworth, J., Shaw, A., Fernandez Crespo, R., Leis, M., Howitt, P., Durkin, M., Neves, A.L. and Darzi, A. 2022. *The National State of Patient Safety: What We Know about Avoidable Harm in England*. Imperial College London.

Institute of Medicine. 2001. *Crossing the Quality Chasm*. National Academies Press.

Kaur, M., De Boer, R.J., Oates, A., Rafferty, J. and Dekker, S. 2019. Restorative just culture: A study of the practical and economic effects of implementing restorative justice in an NHS trust. Presented at ICSC-ESWC 2018 (MATEC Web of Conferences, Vol. 273, Article ID: 01007). https://doi.org/10.1051/matecconf/201927301007

Kirkup, B. 2015. *The Report of the Morecambe Bay Investigation: An Independent Investigation into the Management, Delivery and Outcomes of Care Provided by the Maternity and Neonatal Services at the University Hospitals of Morecambe Bay NHS Foundation Trust from January 2004 to June 2013*. Stationery Office.

Kjeldmand, D. and Holmström, I. 2008. Balint groups as a means to increase job satisfaction and prevent burnout among general practitioners. *The Annals of Family Medicine*, 6(2): 138–145.

Kjeldmand, D., Holmstroem, I. and Rosenqvist, U. 2004. Balint training makes GPs thrive better in their job. *Patient Education and Counseling*, 55(2): 230–235.

Lawrence, G. 1977. *Exploring Individual and Organizational Boundaries: A Tavistock Open Systems Approach*. Tavistock Institute. London.

Lintern, S. 2023. *10 Years On: An Interview with Sir Robert Francis*. Nuffield Trust. https://www.nuffieldtrust.org.uk/news-item/yearsyears10-years-on-an-interview-with-sir-robert-francis

Litz, B.T., Stein, N., Delaney, E., Lebowitz, L., Nash, W.P., Silva, C. and Maguen, S. 2009. Moral injury and moral repair in war veterans: A preliminary model and intervention strategy. *Clinical Psychology Review*, 29(8): 695–706.

Maben, J., Taylor, C., Dawson, J., Leamy, M.C., McCarthy, I., Reynolds, E.F., Ross, S., Shuldham, C., Bennett, L. and Foot, C. 2018. A realist informed mixed-methods evaluation of Schwartz Center Rounds® in England. *Health Services and Delivery Research*, 6(37), 1–260

Malby, B. and Anderson-Wallace, M. 2016. *Healthcare: Managing Complex Relationships.* Emerald Group Publishing Limited.

Martin, G.P., Chew, S. and Dixon-Woods, M. 2021. Uncovering, creating or constructing problems? Enacting a new role to support staff who raise concerns about quality and safety in the English National Health Service. *Health*, 25(6): 757–774.

Martin, G.P., Stanford, S. and Dixon-Woods, M. 2023. A decade after Francis: Is the NHS safer and more open? *BMJ*, 380: 513. https://doi.org/10.1136/bmj.p513

Menzies-Lyth, I. 1960. Social systems as a defence against anxiety: An empirical study of the nursing service of a general hospital. *Human Relations*, 13(2): 95–121.

Miceli, M.P., Near, J.P. and Dworkin, T.M. 2008. *Whistle-Blowing in Organizations.* Psychology Press.

Moreno-Mulet, C., Sansó, N., Carrero-Planells, A., López-Deflory, C., Galiana, L., García-Pazo, P., Borràs-Mateu, M.M. and Miró-Bonet, M. 2021. The impact of the COVID-19 pandemic on ICU healthcare professionals: A mixed methods study. *International Journal of Environmental Research and Public Health*, 18(17): 9243.

Morley, G., Ives, J., Bradbury-Jones, C. and Irvine, F. 2019. What is "moral distress"? A narrative synthesis of the literature. *Nursing Ethics*, 26(3): 646–662. doi: 10.1177/0969733017724354.

Nitsun, M. 2001. Towards a group-analytic approach to individual psychotherapy. *Group Analysis*, 34(4): 473–483.

Obholzer, A. and Roberts, V.R. 1994. *The Unconscious at Work: A Tavistock Approach to Making Sense of Organizational Life.* Routledge.

Ortashi, O., Virdee, J., Hassan, R., Mutrynowski, T and Abu-Zidan, F. 2013. The practice of defensive medicine among hospital doctors in the United Kingdom. *BMC Medical Ethics*, 14: 42. https://doi.org/10.1186/1472-6939-14-42

Point of Care Foundation. n.d. *About Schwartz Rounds.* www.pointofcarefoundation.org.uk/our-programmes/staff-experience/about-schwartz-rounds/

Robert, G., Philippou, J., Leamy, M., Reynolds, E., Ross, S., Bennett, L., Taylor, C., Shuldham, C. and Maben, J. 2017. Exploring the adoption of Schwartz Center Rounds as an organisational innovation to improve staff well-being in England, 2009–2015. *BMJ Open*, 7(1), e014326.

Roberts, J.P. 1982. Foulkes' concept of the matrix. *Group Analysis*, 15(2): 111–126.

Robertson, J.H. and Thomson, A.M. 2014. A phenomenological study of the effects of clinical negligence litigation on midwives in England: The personal perspective. *Midwifery*, 30(3): e121-e130.

Rose, S., Bisson, J. and Wessely, S. 2003. A systematic review of single-session psychological interventions ("debriefing") following trauma. *Psychotherapy and Psychosomatics*, 72(4): 176–184.

Shale, S. 2011. *Moral Leadership in Medicine: Building Ethical Healthcare Organizations*. Cambridge University Press.

Shale, S. 2020. Moral injury and the COVID-19 pandemic: Reframing what it is, who it affects and how care leaders can manage it. *BMJ Leader*, 4(4): 224.

Shale, S. and Anderson-Wallace, M. 2020. *Acting on Concerns and Prosocial Organisational Behaviours*. Occasional paper. London.

Shay, J. 2003. *Odysseus in America: Combat Trauma and the Trials of Homecoming*. Simon and Schuster.

Shay, J. 2010. *Achilles in Vietnam: Combat Trauma and the Undoing of Character*. Simon and Schuster.

Shay, J. 2014. Moral injury. *Psychoanalytic Psychology*, 31(2): 182.

Siegal, G., Mello, M.M. and Studdert, D.M. (2008) Adjudicating severe birth injury claims in Florida and Virginia: The experience of a landmark experiment in personal injury compensation. *American Journal of Law and Medicine*, 34: 489–533.

Skowrońska, J. 2023. *Under the Surface: Unconscious Processes at Helping Institutions*. QMMAC Occasional Paper.

Smith, N. 2008. *I Was Wrong: The Meanings of Apologies*. New York. Cambridge University Press.

Stacey, R.D. 2003. *Complexity and Group Processes: A Radically Social Understanding of Individuals*. Routledge.

Studdert, D.M., Mello, M.M., Sage, W.M., DesRoches, C.M., Peugh, J., Zapert, K. and Brennan, T.A. 2005. Defensive medicine among high-risk specialist physicians in a volatile malpractice environment. *JAMA*, 293(21): 2609–2617. doi: 10.1001/jama.293.21.2609

Thorpe, K.E. 2004. The medical malpractice "crisis": Recent trends and the impact of state tort reforms: Do recent events constitute a crisis or merely the workings of the insurance cycle? *Health Affairs*, 23(Suppl 1): W4–20.

Titcombe, J., Hughes, J. and Anderson-Wallace, M. 2023. *Healing after Healthcare Harm – A Call for Restorative Action*. Harmed Patients Alliance. https://harmedpatientsalliance.org.uk/healing-after-healthcare-harm-a-call-for-restorative-action/

Toker, A., Shvarts, S. and Perry, Z.H. 2004. Clinical guidelines, defensive medicine, and the physician between the two. *American Journal of Otolaryngology*, 25(4): 245–250. doi: 10.1016/j.amjoto.2004.02.002

Van Vliet, K.J. 2008. Shame and resilience in adulthood: A grounded theory study. *Journal of Counseling Psychology*, 55: 233–245. doi: 10.1037/0022-0167.55.2.233

Vandersteegen, T., Marneffe, W., Cleemput, I. and Vereeck, L. 2015. The impact of no-fault compensation on health care expenditures: An empirical study of OECD countries. *Health Policy*, 119: 367–374.

Vincent, C., Stanhope, N. and Crowley-Murphy, M.J. 1999. Reasons for not reporting adverse incidents: An empirical study. *Journal of Evaluation in Clinical Practice*, 5: 13–21.

Vize, R. 2022. Ockenden report exposes failures in leadership, teamwork, and listening to patients. *BMJ*, 376: o860. doi: 10.1136/bmj.o860

Wailling, J., Kooijman, A., Hughes, J. and O'Hara, J.K. 2022. Humanizing harm: Using a restorative approach to heal and learn from adverse events. *Health Expectations,* 25(4): 1192–1199. doi: 10.1111/hex.13478

Wallis, K. 2013. New Zealand's 2005 "no-fault" compensation reforms and medical professional accountability for harm. *The New Zealand Medical Journal,* 126(1371): 33–44.

Waring, J.J. 2005. Beyond blame: Cultural barriers to medical incident reporting. *Social Science & Medicine,* 60: 1927–1935.

Wears, R. and Sutcliffe, K. 2019. *Still Not Safe: Patient Safety and the Middle-Managing of American Medicine.* Oxford University Press.

WHO. 2019. *Patient Safety Fact Sheet.* www.who.int/news-room/fact-sheets/detail/patient-safety

Williams, N. 2018. *Gross Negligence Manslaughter in Healthcare: The Report of a Rapid Policy Review.* Department of Health and Social Care.

Willis, D. 2020. Whorlton Hall, Winterbourne View and Ely Hospital: Learning from failures of care. *Learning Disability Practice,* 23(6). doi: 10.7748/ldp.2020.e2049

11

Understanding Need

━━ Framing ━━

Our aim throughout this book has been to emphasise the importance of understanding the work that needs to be done, before any attempts at improvement are made. As we have discussed elsewhere in this book, a common error that organisations make when seeking to improve or transform is not taking time to understand the nature of their work. Put simply, by failing to question their work, they accept the basic nature of what they currently do - often as the only way - and the consequences of this are profound. They range from making the wrong work more efficient, to reinforcing current structures and models, thereby cementing ways of working that may be unhelpful and inefficient. By not questioning the work, it is easy to make the current better, when what we need to do is something fundamentally different. It also risks creating a level of passive acceptance and can amplify a sense of alienation from the work that needs to be done, or in the alternative encourages a level of complacency, which can equally threaten quality.

In this chapter, we will explore some practical ways to consider understanding needs, drawing on examples from primary care and general practice where a huge amount of healthcare activity happens every day. Our focus on primary care is also partly based on the evidence we have generated from our own practice (Easton & Downham, 2020) but also because research, as mentioned previously, into high performance healthcare systems shows that strong primary care services can make an enormous difference in terms of demand within secondary care services, and in terms of population health within our communities (Baker, 2011; Baker & Denis, 2011).

We also draw on contemporary research and practice drawn from asset-based community development (Russell, 2010, 2017) and co-production (Cahn, 2001; Ostrom, 1996) where the definition of need is seen as a much more co-operated activity, and as a valuable tool for building relationships, social capital and meeting needs more effectively and efficiently.

___

Understanding Need

We start from a position that good service design begins with understanding need, not activity. Yet the process of understanding what is needed, whilst appearing simple, is wrapped in misunderstanding, assumption and complexity (Figure 11.1).

> • Designing the work to do 'what matters' rather than 'what fits'
> • Harnessing the flexibility and creativity in person-centred approaches
> • Understanding the difference between relational and transactional work
> • realising the power of social context

Figure 11.1 Understanding need

Service Design and Exclusion

Good service design involves examining the available data – both quantitatively and qualitatively – but also being totally prepared to question the nature of what is happening right in front us, however challenging that may prove. Frequently, we discover that the data we want is not available and needs collecting. This can be done at various levels and can be immensely valuable in understanding our service interactions with individuals, families, communities, and even across whole populations. Critically, it provides us with the catalyst for curiosity and further inquiry.

As we continue to emphasise throughout this book, as we question the work we must also prepare ourselves and our colleagues for the inevitable challenge to our basic assumptions, and we must be ready to tackle a range of difficult and occasionally uncomfortable issues along the way. This includes addressing historical bias against specific communities and/or people whose needs have been labelled in pejorative ways, often for many years. Our current system involves a wide range of exclusions and prejudices which are not only damaging but ultimately very expensive in terms of end-to-end costs. Many of these issues are firmly embedded in our cultural and societal beliefs, which become expressed in our public services. We routinely misidentify needs based on race, ethnicity, sexual orientation, gender, disability, social class and mental health status. We know that this type of exclusion is particularly prevalent in certain groups who have been consistently marginalised over the decades, and this means that we must be willing to address issues of epistemic exclusion[1] (Dotson, 2014), institutional racism (Kapadia et al., 2022) and medical paternalism (Chin, 2002; Driever et al., 2022).

Understanding need is about giving highly active attention to people who we have misheard, who have been unheard and unseen by our traditional methods of listening, as much as it is about noticing those who are very present, and whose voices are loud and clear. It also involves radically rethinking who should be doing what, and where. It usually comes as something of a shock to practitioners when they realise that for most of the time – excepting the most acute circumstances – their interventions have limited impact, and it is patients, their families, friends and others in their social support networks that really make the difference. This issue is also addressed in Chapter 9, where we explore what we call the "Specialist, Generalist, Citizen Muddle". In short, if we have any chance of providing high-quality services for all, we must be prepared to reconsider the boundaries of traditional practice and think much more carefully and realistically about how good outcomes are produced in the contemporary healthcare setting.

The Social Determinants of Health

There is compelling evidence that social determinants have a huge effect on health (Marmot et al., 2010). According to NHS England only 20% of a person's health outcomes are attributed to the ability to access quality healthcare (NHS England, 2016). This means that the impact of the £150 billion plus of healthcare spending in England is dwarfed by the impact of the social and environmental context. Both the Marmot Review and the Dame Carol Black Review highlighted the huge economic costs of failing to act on the wider determinants of health. As the Rt Hon. Patricia Hewitt articulates in her independent review of the Integrated Care Systems in England (Hewitt, 2023) even before COVID-19, health inequalities were estimated to cost the NHS an extra £4.8 billion a year, society around £31 billion in lost productivity, and between £20 to 32 billion a year in lost tax revenue and benefit payments (Public Health England, 2021). As various policy initiatives point towards more proactive personalised care, and to population health and addressing growing inequalities, designing services and interventions that address the social determinants of health is more important than ever. The evidence is clear: people with no friends, lonely and isolated, are at least as likely to be in poor health as they would be if they were heavy smokers (Holt-Lunstad et al., 2010).

Of course, like so many other areas discussed in this book, there is nothing new in this revelation; indeed the existence of the NHS is – at least in part – a result of this recognition. When social policy expert Sir William Beveridge published his seminal report identifying the so-called "five giants" of Want, Disease, Ignorance, Squalor and Idleness in 1942, he was identifying the social determinants of wellbeing (Beveridge, 1942). Beveridge's "five giants" shaped the modern Welfare State and can be translated in modern parlance as services to support Social Security, Health, Education, Housing and Employment. Of course, what the NHS was set up to tackle in terms of health need in 1948 was vastly different in terms of patterns of disease and illness, and yet the ways in which many services are provided have not evolved at the same pace. Indeed, when Nye Bevan, the Minister responsible for the establishment of the NHS, was challenged about the growing costs, he retorted that people should not be worried, as in years to come the cost of healthcare would have diminished dramatically as the population would have become much healthier because of the services provided by the NHS.

Life and Social Contextual Pressures

To be clear on terminology, from this point onwards, we will refer to social determinants as life or social context pressures as this feels like a more accurate reflection of what we are discussing. Living life with social contextual pressure does not necessarily mean you are involved with statutory services – indeed those people are just a small minority. This means that the extent of need in the populace is hugely underestimated, especially if we only consider those people who can be easily identified through activity. Dahlgren and Whitehead (2021) illustrate the multiple influences on a person's health of education, living and working conditions, unemployment, housing, social and community networks, individual lifestyle factors and a wide range of general socio-economic, cultural, and environmental conditions. At one level this can appear overwhelming to practitioners, and it is not surprising that those working in primary care become concerned about the impact on their workloads as they try to consider how best to respond to the myriad complexity that these conditions bring. But the good news is that there are ways of tackling these issues; they have a long history of success, and the principles can be applied if people are willing to change the way that they work.

Person and Community Centred Approaches

In the English NHS, Tameside and Glossop's Person and Community Centred Approaches team have been working with primary care general practices to support them in understanding the practical implications of these social contextual pressures. Part of this approach has been to create a three-level lens to broadly segment need. The intention of this work was to stimulate conversations around new models of care and bring to life what those working in primary care have instinctively known for decades. Figure 11.2 features the outputs from a GP-led study of over 2000 consultations (telephone and face to face). It details GP-led segmentation from over ten practices, each looking at a week of consulting patterns. It details the proportion of patients likely to be under social contextual pressure.

The three context segments are:

- Stable (default to if context not known) – this means that the person is coping in a stable life context and has an identifiable network of support
- Under pressure – this means that the person has one or more social and environmental stressors relating to housing, no work or precarious employment, financial worries, relationship difficulties, caring duties and/or is lonely
- Turbulent – this means that the person has severe issues associated with ongoing mental health problems, severe social stressors, drug and/or alcohol misuse, and is a frequent user of services (health, social care, criminal justice, police etc.)

Contextual Pressure

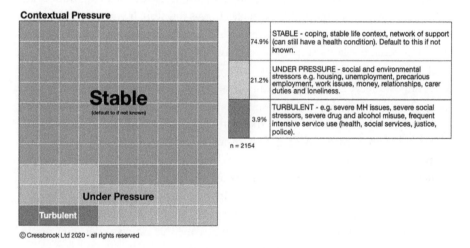

Figure 11.2 Contextual pressure in general practice

This data tells us that, in their GP's view, 25% of all the patients that attended in that week are experiencing social contextual pressure. Almost 4% of them experience this to an extraordinarily elevated level of turbulence. In other words, life is not easy at all. For most these "social stressors" relate to caring duties, loneliness, relationships, housing, precarious employment and financial worries. For a small proportion of that 25%, the level of turbulence in their lives is very severe. This means they are known to the statutory services and regularly access the health, social care and criminal justice systems. It is important to say that being under pressure is not just about socio-economic factors – you can of course be financially secure but isolated or in a problematic relationship. It is also not just about health. Similarly, you can have a significant health condition, but still be stable in your life context. This means that clinical acuity does not always correlate directly with need.

While most GPs do not have this data to hand, they most certainly will have observed it in their everyday practice. But just because we know this, it does not mean we design services with this in mind. In fact, talking to GPs around the country, despite moves towards approaches which take account of the social contextual pressures – such as social prescribing – general practice often struggles to help people with needs outside the linear bio-medical, and/or to have significant impact on those conditions that have a large life context or lifestyle component.

It's About Life, not Lifestyle

As the Marmot Strategic Review of Health Inequalities report makes clear, the social context of your life is about so much more than just lifestyle choices (Marmot et al., 2010). It is often about the ability to make choices full stop. If you are living under severe life context pressure – whether you are lonely, in poor housing, in a problematic or violent relationship, or if you have precarious employment, or a mix of all of these – making positive choices about your health may be extremely difficult, if not impossible. For example, conditions such as type 2 diabetes are considered to have a significant "lifestyle" component. Education is therefore often considered to be a key intervention. GPs know that patients need to be in the "right place" to hear and act upon their advice and these social contextual pressures clearly limit the effectiveness of their interventions. This does not of course take in account the challenges that many may have in accessing and affording a so-called "healthy diet". If we then consider the 4% who are living in a turbulent state and arguably the 21% under some form of contextual pressure, their ability to interact with services becomes even more complex. Put simply, there is no way that our current system of primary care can serve these people well.

There are at least two defining characteristics that make our current model of care less effective at helping people under this type of contextual life pressure. The first is that services are hugely fragmented. Care is split into small chunks and delivered by countless professionals and services. This makes it hugely difficult to maintain a relationship with a patient or hold their context (Davis, 2016). Meeting their healing, caring and biographical domains of practice becomes a huge challenge. The second is that the health system is predicated on a deficit model, rather than one that is asset based. In other words, as we touched on in Chapter 9, we operate a model that concentrates on understanding what makes you ill, rather than what makes you healthy.

There is much debate about whether health services – such as a general practice – should aim to meet what are social needs, but this is a fruitless argument because patients use the services anyway. Often a social need is presented as a health condition with a genuine medical presentation and general practice is also one of the last remaining places people can get help without significant barriers to entry. General practitioners are also increasingly the gatekeepers to other services. The second reason is that not

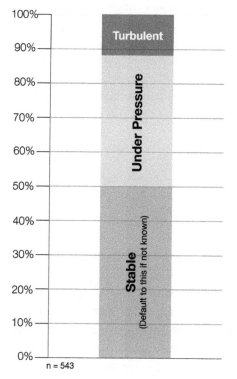

Figure 11.3 Social context pressure (high attenders)

helping with underlying contextual pressures can make health conditions much worse. People decline in their wellbeing and eventually present themselves with conditions that are more complex and developed, creating more work, not less. To illustrate this, when GPs applied the same segmentation to high attending patients within the same group of practices, the proportion grew to 50% of patients that were "under pressure" or "turbulent" in context – as can be seen in Figure 11.3.

It is worth noting that this group of 543 high attending patients, from over ten practices, accounted for 12,910 face to face or telephone consultations over the previous year. The argument here is that the extent of social context pressure should have as much bearing on the service design as acuity or a specific health condition. It heavily shapes how we help people. Despite this most GP services are designed around the bio-medical, even though at least one in four patients have broader needs that are likely to undermine traditional health interventions.

While we are discussing this through the lens of general practice, the message is certainly applicable in more specialist settings. As more and more interventions are moved to day case, and there is a greater reliance on outpatient clinics and a drive to move diagnostics and some therapies into home settings, an understanding of context matters. The level of contextual pressure a patient is under will determine the success of these things for individual patients and should be at the centre of a clinician's and service's thinking when designing and using pathways.

Multiple handoffs between services and professionals make understanding life context even more difficult. Information and trust fall between the cracks of multiple services creating additional Failure Demand. Defragmenting (simplifying) the response to need is key. This requires much more than common integration activities of co-location, information sharing and single points of access. This is discussed in further detail in Chapter 8.

How Much Work Is There to Do?

As has been discussed in Chapter 5, improvement work usually starts with some form of demand analysis. How can you improve a service without knowing how much work it has to do? Many organisations skip this critical step, preferring to jump straight into analysing their activity data to answer this question. But activity data only tells you who you let in, rather than who *needed* the service. If you are incredibly lucky, these things may be the same, but in most cases they are not. Activity data commonly also has a lag in it. It tells you when someone presented or had an intervention, but it does not tell you when the need arose. Also, understanding demand as a simple number is also not enough. We need to understand the nature of the work to design services to meet that need. Demand also only reduces if you meet it, not manage it – and in healthcare that starts with responding to need. We are explicitly using the word "design" as this is a very deliberate and purposeful process, and although even the most carefully designed services can still struggle to keep pace with rapidly changing needs, it is much better than simplistic responses based on the firefighting pressures that drive much service improvement.

Viewing the Work Differently

A great deal of demand data that is available within healthcare settings is based around what are often described as labelled needs (Davis, 2016). These labelled needs tend to mirror the current system design, structures and response, and people need to fit those categories to be able to access the service. This has two effects, firstly people adapt their needs to fit the label and secondly it simply reinforces the current structures. If we fail to do this then we risk making the wrong thing righter; that is to say improving a way of working that is still not likely to meet the needs of those who use it.

A practical example of this would be to look at the "front door" of most healthcare systems – called primary care and specifically general practice in the English NHS.

Looking at this common first point of access can give us important insights beyond primary care and into the pressures more specialist secondary care hospital settings face. Starting from the position of needing a new view, we advocate keeping things simple. Whilst there are many ways to categorise healthcare work we will use two broad archetypes, which can be particularly useful when beginning this journey. We appreciate this is an oversimplification but for the purposes of illustration we are taking the risk.

In the first category, we consider the linear work of primary care. These are process-driven bio-medical responses to helping people for which the current system is designed. Examples are a diagnostic test, an onward referral to a clinical specialist or medical assessment, or surgical intervention in a secondary care environment. This work can be highly technical in nature and a successful outcome in the process is reliant on several things coming together with high reliability. It tends to be highly specified in form and timing. This is sometimes described as transactional work and much service commissioning assumes the work in primary care is linear in nature.

Characteristics of linear work:

- Highly defined in process
- Specified in nature, entry criteria and timing
- Transactional relationships between the various parts of the process
- High degree of certainty and reliability of interventions and timing define outcomes
- Can be hugely technical in nature (such as a surgical intervention)
- Outcomes and standards can be easily defined
- Pathways and processes are split amongst functionally specialised providers, teams and professionals
- Market and financial incentives are used as management tools
- The life context of the patient does not limit the outcomes of the intervention in the short and medium term
- Delivered through hierarchical structures
- Improved through QI techniques (process mapping and waste identification)

The second category of work is what might be considered more relational. This is work where the response is concerned with factors outside the biomedical sphere, including the person's environment and social circumstances. An example would be helping someone living with type 2 diabetes or trying to slow the disease progression of someone living with chronic respiratory problems. This work tends to be characterised as involving a person's life and lifestyle – or more accurately how they are positioned in a network of relationships and the degree of social contextual pressure they experience.

Characteristics of relational work:

- System designed to be able to iteratively help someone (to loop and try again multiple times)
- Adopt asset-based starting points with patients – focusing on what makes you well vs what makes you ill
- High degree of flexibility to help the patient "do what matters" to them and help them exercise more agency in their own lives and relationships (Marmot et al., 2010)
- High degree of continuity avoiding deferring and referring where possible
- Emphasis on helping the patient create a support network and sense of purpose
- Time for professionals to create trust and build relationships
- Long-term funding arrangements
- Enabled through network-based structures
- Improved through systems thinking

Even though these are crude distinctions, you need to organise and design services differently to meet the needs of those involved differently, depending on which is dominant or in the foreground at any given time.

Figure 11.4 illustrates the split of these two work categories as seen by a typical general practice over a week. This practice was in a relatively deprived urban area. Looking at the 262 consultations analysed, the white represents patients who required no further action, the light grey represents patients who needed a linear response and the dark grey represents patients who needed a relational response. It shows that 29% of patients required no follow-up at all, 50% required a classic

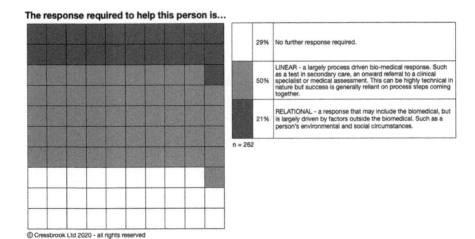

The response required to help this person is...

29%	No further response required.
50%	LINEAR - a largely process driven bio-medical response. Such as a test in secondary care, an onward referral to a clinical specialist or medical assessment. This can be highly technical in nature but success is generally reliant on process steps coming together.
21%	RELATIONAL - a response that may include the biomedical, but is largely driven by factors outside the biomedical. Such as a person's environmental and social circumstances.

n = 262

Figure 11.4   Linear and relational responses

The response required to help this group of high attending patients

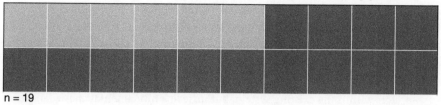

n = 19

	32 %	LINEAR - a largely process driven bio-medical response. Such as a test in secondary care, an onward referral to a clinical specialist or medical assessment. This can be highly technical in nature but success is generally reliant on process steps coming together.
	68 %	RELATIONAL - a response that may include the biomedical, but is largely driven by factors outside the biomedical. Such as a person's environmental and social circumstances.

Figure 11.5   Linear and relational - high attenders

bio-medical response – which the service is designed and run to do – and a very considerable 21% of people required a relational response – which it is not.

As illustrated in Figure 11.5, this plays out when you use the same analysis to look at people who attend general practice frequently. The practice reviewed 19 people who they categorised in this way. These people accounted for 1165 practice interactions (both face to face and teleconsultations) and a minimum of 265 secondary care interactions in the previous year. Of these 19 people, 68% required a predominantly relational response to help them. People who attend services frequently, especially over a long, multi-year period, in the majority do not present with linear biomedical issues.

To meet this demand, a system needs a model that is capable of relational work. Small steps like social prescribing can be helpful, but given the proportions, it is in a practice's best interest to shift to a much more relational model if it wants to respond to the presenting needs of the local population. At regional and policy level, if the NHS is ever to meet its self-identified targets of reducing demands on secondary care, greater anticipatory care, reducing health inequalities and improving long-term conditions, then it must get much better at this work, and the first step is to stop assuming all the work is linear.

General practice is traditionally a trusted institution in many communities, although it is fair to say that recently this has come under significant pressure. People come regardless of whether their need is health or social. We argue it should not be up to the public to try and work out if their need fits the correct box. In some places, the changes are happening already. Changes to models such as longer and more flexible appointment lengths, group-based consultations, group-based peer support groups, practice community champions, in-house mental health provision, direct messaging, talking groups, links to schools, walking groups and lunch groups are all helping practices help their patients in diverse ways.

Although these issues often manifest in general practice, they cannot be tackled by general practice alone. Person-centred approaches are at their best where entire health and care systems consider these approaches a priority and collaborate to respond to need in a coordinated manner. This is not about the delivery of new services within the existing system, but instead a fundamental change in basic assumptions that puts all the services delivered by health and care firmly in the frame of the life context of the person receiving them. We should not underestimate the scale of this challenge, but nor should we shy away from it.

Social Prescribing and Asset-Based Approaches

Social prescribing has been described as a key component of a universal approach to personalised care and is defined as an approach that connects people to activities, groups, and services in their community to meet the practical, social and emotional needs that affect their health and wellbeing (NHS England, 2016).

Social prescribing is said to be an all-age, entire population approach that works particularly well for people who:

- have one or more long-term conditions
- need support with low level mental health issues
- are lonely or isolated
- have complex social needs which affect their wellbeing.

(Adapted from Dayson & Bashir, 2014)

Some argue that this increasingly popular idea is merely an extension of the traditional narrow perspective that dominates healthcare services and is motivated by an attempt to shift the burden of demand in general practice elsewhere, rather than as a genuine response to meeting the needs of people living with social context pressures. Malby et al. (2019) discuss this in detail and argue however that when social prescribing is done well, it can have particularly important multiplier effects on family and friends. They cite work in the Netherlands, that shows that a third of patients who were "socially prescribed" go on to become volunteers and note the beginning of similar patterns in projects studied in the UK. They advise that anyone considering social prescribing as a solution should first ask themselves eight core questions to explore purpose, measurement, status, language, method, scale, costs and significance – see Figure 11.6.

1. Is social prescribing about shifting the burden, or is it about meeting complex needs? (purpose)
2. Should it be about people living well, or about reducing the burden on A&E, or on GP practices? (measurement)
3. Should it be carried out by professionals or volunteers? (status)
4. Should it be based on a national formula or on an emerging face-to-face relationship? (method)
5. Should it describe the new role as social prescribers or community connectors? (language)
6. What scale should it be based upon? (size)
7. How should we pay for it? (costs)
8. Does this amount to a new model of care?

(Adapted from Malby et al., 2019)

Figure 11.6 Social prescribing eight core questions (adapted from Malby et al., 2019)

Malby et al. (2019) however ask whether the term "social prescribing" implies too close a relationship with the medical model, which is the very idea that the approach is attempting to escape from. Sceptics might go further and argue that social prescribing simply mirrors a traditionally myopic view of healthcare, driven by the legacy of clinical hierarchy, medical paternalism and the social status of doctors. Russell (2017) argues that the shortcomings of social prescribing are inevitable and that the prime reason for this is that too much emphasis and expectation is being placed on general practice and third sector organisations, and not enough support and animation are being offered to the associational life of communities themselves. Others support this argument and suggest that we need to be more cognisant of the fact that our communities are rich with assets that can support people with their health and wellbeing – that can be accessed without the need for referral to a link worker, care navigator or social prescriber (Easton & Downham, 2020; Kretzmann et al., 2005).

Asset-based community development approaches are based on the fundamental tenet that every community has "assets" in a variety of domains, including people, associations, institutions, physical space, exchanges and culture. They are built on the goal of fostering local assets and capabilities. Citing a significant body of literature, Malby et al. (2019) explain that "from an asset-based approach, community begins and ends with people, and the social values that shape on the ground experience and organizational practices" (p. 62). A place-based approach to health and wellbeing however potentially provides the opportunity to create a stronger link between formal health and care services and these community assets. General practices undoubtedly have a role in connecting people and triggering further networks, but it is communities, rather than practices, that give people the network and sense of purpose that enable them to help themselves. If you look under the skin of one of the most celebrated general practice models in the UK, the Bromley-by-Bow Health Living Centre, it was a community resource before it became a general practice.

The Peckham Experiment

Yet again we are reminded that in many ways these ideas are not new. In 1926, a group of 30 laypeople from the community and two doctors – Dr Scott Williamson and Dr Innes Pearce – opened a subscription-based "family club" in a small, terraced house in Peckham. Their aim was to understand what caused "health" and the Peckham experiment was established (Pearce & Crocker, 2013). The experiment adopted a fascinating approach that relied on a high degree of self-organisation, where people were encouraged to use the family club to do what they wanted, whenever they wanted, supported and encouraged by the two doctors. By 1929 the family club had 112 families – for it was the family, and their context, not the individual that was the unit of interest[2] – and by 1936 a new purpose-built "health centre" for 2000 families had been constructed including a swimming pool, gym, dance hall, library and cafe – which incidentally was supplied by their own organic farm in Kent. The focus of all the facilities was social connection and cohesion, and the centre was seen as a study of the "living structure" of society. The 1930s was a decade of huge social upheaval and experimentation. The Great Depression ushered in an age of uncertainty and fear and destroyed orthodox beliefs in social, political and economic order. Keynesian economic theories had challenged orthodox proponents of free trade and market equilibrium, and there was significant experimentation in the fields of social welfare and health. The movement was given a sense of urgency by the data revealed by the experiment. Only 10% of the membership could be described as in full health; 30% of members were ill, while 60% were to some extent "compromised" by symptoms they often didn't even realise they had. The "health centre" paid particular attention to pre and antenatal care, early years development as well as regular health monitoring, but its real focus was not on medical symptoms, but what we now describe as the social determinants of health. The development of the centre was interrupted by World War 2, and then in the post-war period – despite the attempts to restart the centre by its users – the model was not considered to fit well with the new National Health Service, which saw a strong desire for centralisation and regulation, with the predomination of medical general practice and acute secondary / specialist care facilities – i.e. hospitals. With no funds to support its ongoing work, the Peckham Experiment finally ended in 1950.

We mention this example for three main reasons. Firstly, to illustrate an example of early co-production – this was a club with members who participated, they were not the recipients of charity or state largesse. Secondly, the level of self-organisation was high – people did what they wanted, when they wanted, admittedly within the confines of a given structure. Finally, the experiment was focused firmly on the relational – families as the primary unit, and families connecting with other families to create community.

Many contend that more widely adopted strategies that emphasise collectivism, collaboration and coproduction can aid in our understanding of the hidden assets in local communities and organisations and in our ability to work imaginatively with people, groups and front line staff to address the wider determinants of health (Ganz et al., 2010; Kimberlee, 2013). The question of whether these approaches can become more than another policy rhetoric with no serious intent to encourage a different type of organisational and grassroots change is uncertain (Malby et al., 2019).

Illness and the Socio-Cultural – Trauma-Informed Care

In a world where social isolation, cultural alienation, loneliness, poverty and growing health inequalities are present, another important consideration is the extent to which active pathology should be understood and reframed in socio-cultural rather than bio-medical terms. We recognise that this is a crude distinction but for the sake of illustration we will take the risk.

Lifetime traumatic events are known to have a detrimental long-term impact on both mental and physical health. Epidemiological and biomedical evidence link adverse childhood experiences (ACEs) with health-harming behaviours and the development of non-communicable disease in adults (Bellis et al., 2014). Higher rates of chronic diseases, medically unexplained symptoms and unhealthy substance use are strongly associated with ACEs, and it is well known that groups who experience elevated levels of health disparity often have much higher rates of exposure to these adverse experiences. Studies conducted over the past two decades show that adult health profiles relate to childhood stressors such as parental substance misuse, incarceration and domestic violence, and that ACEs have been related to increased propensity for substance use (alcohol, tobacco and drugs), anti-social behaviour, and ultimately development of cardiovascular disease, cancer, chronic lung disease and diabetes (Anda et al., 2006; Felitti et al., 2019). Work from the USA also identified strong relationships between ACEs and adult obesity (Bellis et al., 2014). Childhood trauma can have effects that can last until adolescence and into adulthood (Wilkinson, 2018). Significantly, research has shown that the number of stressors (i.e., the ACE count) is a significant predictor of bad mental health and, as a result, poor health outcomes over the course of a person's life. Moreover, growing up with many stressors is linked to future unwanted pregnancies, as well as being a perpetrator or victim of violence, including intimate partner abuse. Together, these sexual and aggressive behaviours produce a mechanism for the transmission of ACEs and their negative health effects between generations (Dietz et al., 1999; Whitfield et al., 2003).

In response to an increasing understanding of these issues, it is argued that service and practice solutions must be created to recognise and address the experience of complex trauma in the lives of the individuals with whom they make contact. The underlying premise of trauma-informed care is that it combines relational and strengths-based approaches of working to address the impact of trauma, despite the lack of agreement on a definition that specifies its precise nature (Wilkinson, 2018).

A Trauma-Informed Primary Care Response

At the Southcentral Foundation in Alaska (also referred to in Chapters 3 and 9) it was recognised that a sizable proportion of the indigenous population were living life with elevated levels of chronic illness. This included alarming levels of mental health difficulties, alcohol and drug misuse and completed suicide in young men. The history and experiences of the native Alaskan population – like many indigenous groups around the world – have been brutal. The effects of colonisation and the disease that followed decimated communities, and years of oppression and maltreatment engendered a sense of cultural alienation and epistemic exclusion. The level of intergenerational trauma is profound.

A novel approach to improving physical health by helping adults to heal from trauma through the generations was adopted. Several culturally sensitive trauma-informed Family Wellness Warrior (FWW) programmes were developed to specifically address these issues, which were evaluated based on the hypothesis that participation in them could reverse the negative health effects of adverse experiences. The FWW programme includes a variety of methods intended to support persons affected by violence and heal trauma. To comprehend their own experiences, the origins of abuse, and how to break the cycle, participants work in groups. They learn how previous wrongdoing, rage and fear affect how they interact with others and how the actions and decisions of the following generation frequently reflect what they have witnessed and heard. Participants begin by sharing their stories to understand and heal themselves. Gaining self-confidence and self-esteem because of this healing enables individuals to forge meaningful connections. Lastly, they can help others and can draw on their first-hand experiences to aid in others' healing. The FWW programme is said to differ from many trauma-informed approaches because it is created and led by Alaskan natives, is culturally and spirituality rooted, and uses peer leaders and modelling rather than clinical hierarchy.

A propensity-matched retrospective cohort study compared post-programme healthcare utilisation changes for 90 participants to healthcare utilisation changes for a 90-person comparison group. All cohort members were Alaskans. The study indicated that the FWW programme significantly reduced emergency department and substance use visits by 55% and 79% respectively. In addition, evaluation data showed significant reductions in unhealthy substance use, trauma symptomology, depression and anxiety. For example, 67% of men and 71% of women who attended the programmes showed a reduction in depression.

Conclusion – Not Just a Healthcare Problem

In this chapter we have considered the challenges associated with understanding need, with a particular focus on primary care and general practice. This focus was in part to enable us to draw upon our own practice experience and research but also because strong primary care provision is seen as central to creating high-performing healthcare systems (Baker & Denis, 2011).

We have shown how poorly healthcare often responds to the *actual needs* of a considerable proportion of people who use those services, and we have considered the Failure Demand – the extra work that is generated by the way we organise the work – that is created as a result. It is important to stress that our critique is not a reflection on the dedicated practitioners who work within these services; it is an indictment of the approach of the broader system of public services to understanding need. The problem of mis-identifying need and then organising services doing "the wrong work" is certainly not confined to healthcare – it is a problem that afflicts many public services.

For instance, policing has been under a deal of criticism recently for not providing for the needs of the community it is supposed to serve. Police officers have been said to solve an exceedingly small percentage of crimes. In England and Wales it has been reported that in 2021, 98.7% of rapes and 19 out of every 20 burglaries and violent offences went unsolved. Four out of every ten cases were closed without identifying a suspect (The Telegraph, 2022; The Times, 2022). It has been argued that the police simply do not deal with criminality in most cases, instead they spend a great deal of time handling societal problems caused by people who are disproportionately poor and/or in need of mental health care (Jones, 2023). But alternative options do exist. For example, a group of health professionals in Denver respond to trespassing and mental health emergencies involving non-violent, vulnerable people. These are cases that armed police have previously handled. Or consider the Oregon city of Eugene, where a team of medics and experienced crisis workers have been addressing issues such as welfare visits, disorientated people and those in mental health crisis, all of which had previously been handled by armed police units. The team handled 20% of all calls to the city's public safety communication centre in 2022, yet only 301 of the 22,000 calls they handled required police back-up assistance (CAHOOTS Program Analysis, 2021).

What these services demonstrate is an understanding of actual need – and they do so based on the data that is clearly available both through the real demands placed on services every day and based on the lived experience of professionals and citizens. The aim is not to shift the burden of work from one service to another, it is to respond to people's real needs – and to meet them as far as is possible. Surely this is a better way to plan for an uncertain future than clinging to outmoded and costly versions of services that dominate current practice by habit and tradition.

Acknowledgements

We would like to thank Chris Easton for his support and contribution in shaping the thinking and data used to help form this chapter.

Notes

1 Epistemic exclusion questions normative beliefs about what forms of knowledge (epistemology) are valued and which producers of knowledge are deemed legitimate.
2 This family focus offers strong similarities to the much-heralded Family Health System – Community Health Worker model we explored in Chapter 8.

References

Anda, R.F., Felitti, V.J., Bremner, J.D., Walker, J.D., Whitfield, C.H., Perry, B.D., Dube, S.R. and Giles, W.H. 2006. The enduring effects of abuse and related adverse experiences in childhood: A convergence of evidence from neurobiology and epidemiology. *European Archives of Psychiatry and Clinical Neuroscience*, 256: 174–186.

Baker, G. 2011. *The Roles of Leaders in High-Performing Health Care Systems*. The King's Fund.

Baker, G. and Denis, J. 2011. *A Comparative Study of Three Transformative Healthcare Systems with Lessons for Canada*. Canadian Health Services Research Foundation, Toronto, Ontario.

Bellis, M.A., Hughes, K., Leckenby, N., Perkins, C. and Lowey, H. 2014. National household survey of adverse childhood experiences and their relationship with resilience to health-harming behaviors in England. *BMC Medicine*, 12(72). https://doi.org/10.1186/1741-7015-12-72

Beveridge, S.W. 1942. *Report on Social Insurance and Allied Services*. para 305, Cmd. 6404.

Cahn, E. 2001. *No More Throwaway People: The Co-Production Imperative*. Essential Books.

CAHOOTS Program Analysis. 2021. *Update (2022) Eugene Police Department Crime Analysis.* www.eugene-or.gov/4508/CAHOOTS

Chin, J.J. 2002. Doctor–patient relationship: From medical paternalism to enhanced autonomy. *Singapore Medical Journal*, 43(3): 152–155.

Dahlgren, G. and Whitehead, M. 2021. The Dahlgren-Whitehead model of health determinants: 30 years on and still chasing rainbows. *Public Health*, 199: 20–24.

Davis, R. 2016. *Responsibility and Public Services.* Triarchy Press.

Dayson, C. and Bashir, N. 2014. *The Social and Economic Impact of the Rotherham Social Prescribing Pilot.* Sheffield Hallam University.

Dietz, P.M., Spitz, A.M., Anda, R.F., Williamson, D.F., McMahon, P.M., Santelli, J.S., Nordenberg, D.F., Felitti, V.J. and Kendrick, J.S. 1999. Unintended pregnancy among adult women exposed to abuse or household dysfunction during their childhood. *JAMA*, 282: 1359–1364.

Dotson, K. 2014. Conceptualizing epistemic oppression. *Social Epistemology*, 28(2): 115–138.

Driever, E.M., Tolhuizen, I.M., Duvivier, R.J., Stiggelbout, A.M. and Brand, P.L.P. 2022. Why do medical residents prefer paternalistic decision making? An interview study. *BMC Medical Education*, 22(155). https://doi.org/10.1186/s12909-022-03203-2

Easton, C. and Downham, N. 2020. *The Reality of Patient Social Context in General Practice: The Case for Person and Community Centred Service Design.* www.cressbrookltd.co.uk/the-reality-of-social-context-gp/

Felitti, V.J., Anda, R.F., Nordenberg, D., Williamson, D.F., Spitz, A.M., Edwards, V., Koss, M.P. and Marks, J.S. 2019. Relationship of childhood abuse and household dysfunction to many of the leading causes of death in adults: The adverse childhood experiences (ACE) study. *American Journal of Preventive Medicine*, 14(4): 245–258.

Ganz, M., Nohria, N. and Khurana, R. 2010. Leading change. In *Handbook of Leadership Theory and Practice: A Harvard Business School Centennial Colloquium*, pp. 1–42. Harvard Business Press.

Hewitt, P. 2023. *The Hewitt Review: An Independent Review of Integrated Care Systems.* Department of Health and Social Care.

Holt-Lunstad, J., Smith, T.B. and Bradley Layton, J. 2010. Social relationships and mortality risk: A meta-analytic review. *PLoS Medicine*, 7(7): e1000316.

Jones, O. 2023. Scrapping the Met isn't enough: There are radical – and proven – alternatives. *The Guardian.* www.theguardian.com/commentisfree/2023/mar/23/met-police-uk-radical-alternatives-policing

Kapadia, D., Zhang, J., Salway, S., Nazroo, J., Booth, A., Villarroel-Williams, N., Becares, L. and Esmail, A. 2022. *Ethnic Inequalities in Healthcare: A Rapid Evidence Review.* www.nhsrho.org/publications/ethnic-inequalities-in-healthcare-a-rapid-evidence-review/

Kimberlee, R.H. (2013) *Developing a Social Prescribing Approach for Bristol.* University of the West of England. http://eprints.uwe.ac.uk/23221/1/Social%20Prescribing%20Report-final.pdf

Kretzmann, J.P., McKnight, J. and Puntenney, D. 2005. *Discovering Community Power: A Guide to Mobilizing Local Assets and Your Organization's Capacity*. Asset-Based Community Development Institute, School of Education and Social Policy, Northwestern University.

Malby, R., Boyle, D., Wildman, J., Omar, B.S. and Smith, S. 2019. *The Asset Based Health Inquiry: How Best to Develop Social Prescribing*. London South Bank University.

Marmot, M., Allen, J., Goldblatt, P., Boyce, T., McNeish, D., Grady, M. and Geddes, I. 2010. *The Marmot Review: Fair Society, Healthy Lives. The Strategic Review of Health Inequalities in England Post-2010*. The Stationery Office.

NHS England. 2016. *General Practice Forward View*. www.england.nhs.uk/wp-content/uploads/2016/04/gpfv.pdf

Ostrom, E. 1996. Crossing the great divide: Coproduction, synergy, and development. *World Development*, 24(6): 1073–1087.

Pearse, I.H. and Crocker, L.H. 2013. *The Peckham Experiment: A Study of the Living Structure of Society*. Routledge.

Public Health England. 2021. *Inclusion and Sustainable Economies: Leaving No One Behind*. Public Health England.

Russell, C. 2010. Making the case for an asset-based community development (ABCD) approach to probation: From reformation to transformation. *Irish Probation Journal*, 7: 119–131.

Russell, C. 2017. *Social Prescribing, A Panacea or Another Top-Down Programme? Part 1*. ABCD Thought Leadership Blog. www.nurturedevelopment.org/blog/abcd-approach/social-prescribing-panacea-another-top-programme-part-1/

The Telegraph. 2022. Record low of just 5.8% of crimes solved. www.telegraph.co.uk/news/2022/04/28/record-number-crimes-go-unsolved/

The Times. 2022. Burglars go unpunished with only 5% of cases solved. www.thetimes.co.uk/article/burglars-go-unpunished-with-only-5-of-cases-solved-sk0p0wjmv

Whitfield, C.L., Anda, R.F., Dube, S.R. and Felitti, V.J. 2003. Violent childhood experiences and the risk of intimate partner violence in adults: Assessment in a large health maintenance organization. *Journal of Interpersonal Violence*, 18: 166–185.

Wilkinson, J. 2018. *Developing and Leading Trauma-Informed Practice*. Research in Practice.

Conclusion

In the first part of this book, we explored the history of quality improvement in healthcare, drawing on literature to tell the story of healthcare improvement and explore its roots in industrial and modern management thinking. By focusing on the key actors in the story, we traced the evolution of the ideas and explored how they were introduced, used and assimilated in the culture of the NHS. We examined how we understand notions of "culture" and how these understandings might apply in a healthcare context. We also proposed that a strong appreciation of the socio-cultural dimensions of improvement work is critical when it comes to designing, evaluating and sustaining intervention. We took a "deep dive" into some of the technical dimensions of quality thinking, with a strong focus on understanding variation, demand, capacity and utilisation. In this domain, we specifically emphasised the importance of working with the tensions and dilemmas created when considering variation. They are not resolvable per se, and yet huge gains can be made by thinking about how the tensions are enacted in context. We emphasised the critical importance of raising questions about how much work there is to do; and how we might know whether it is the "right work" to begin with *before* we try to improve it.

We then set out a pragmatic framework for analysis of quality problems in healthcare, focusing on identifying and reducing "Failure Demand" – the immense demands placed on services due to failings of the service and wider system itself – rather than by the demand generated by accurately and flexibly understanding and meeting the needs of the populace. In the final part of the book, we outline four domains where we think practical action can be taken to reduce Failure Demand and improve quality in contemporary care settings. Whilst we completely accept that there are many ways in which we could have categorised these dimensions – indeed they have developed a great deal in our own minds over time – we also take a pragmatic view that they serve a purpose and are good enough for now, and will certainly evolve in the future.

Defragmenting to Integrate

This domain highlights how many services are "fragmented by design" in that they have been built with a remarkable number of transitions. These points of "de-coupling" represent both risk and cost and are often designed to suit service providers or the professionals, with limited if any consideration of the needs of the citizen or end user. To make it worse, a common response to this problem is to overlay another service on top of the existing service to try to mitigate the risk. Inadvertently, this frequently adds extra complication and cost in the process. We propose that an alternative approach is to fundamentally question and reframe how the work is done by actively Defragmenting to Integrate. Frequently, this means rethinking how, by whom and where the work is done and links firmly to our second category.

Avoiding the Specialist, Generalist, Citizen Muddle

This domain tackles the thorny issue of what work is best done by whom, and in what context. Untangling the Specialist, Generalist and Citizen Muddle relies on challenging a great deal of the traditional wisdom about service design and provision, including questioning our taken-for-granted assumptions about professional hierarchies and power structures, and promoting alternative approaches to knowledge equity and sharing responsibility and risk. This often involves giving up "protected territory" and recognising the huge resources that lie within local communities. This radical rethink of the traditional power dynamic between those who give and receive services can enable dramatic strides towards more equal relationships, which can in our view bring about very meaningful long-term improvements in quality. It also relies on a much greater flexibility to identify and respond to need, and being willing to abandon many of the unhelpful and exclusive categories of labelling need.

Understanding Need

This domain relates to how services often deliver services based on labelled needs (i.e. predefined narrow categories) rather than based on a deeper understanding of population needs as expressed within local communities. We also consider the massive effect of the social determinants of health in shaping need, which will inevitably completely overwhelm the health system's attempts to respond. This includes a great deal of activity, which serves neither professionals nor citizens, and is hungry in terms of demand for precious resources. Where demand then overwhelms the service's ability to respond, barriers to entry are often put in place, which can drive need underground. At worst this can lead to a vast cadre of people with unmet needs, with an attendant amplification of problems in the wider network of public services. The response we propose involves a much more flexible approach to services – particularly in primary care – and a recalibration of the system understanding to low- to medium-level acuity and a strong recognition of the influence of social determinants of health.

Supporting Human Systems at Work

This final domain recognises the need for a critical appreciation of the unique moral, ethical and psychological conditions present within healthcare, and the effects when these dimensions are not carefully considered in systemic design. Healthcare is an intensely human business, which deals with people in extreme and disturbing times in their lives. It also supports people over a lifetime, and the people who work within it are often committed to it for their lifetimes too. This creates a relationship over time, which is especially important to recognise if healthcare wants to think about long-term impact on staff and on citizens, many of whom are one and the same. Our proposition in this category is that much greater attention needs to be given to these complex circumstances, and critically to build a strong and consistent moral and ethical framework to support professionals and citizens throughout their long-term relationship to healthcare. This involves developing a strong and fair system that governs the daily workings of healthcare, but also having a supportive, compassionate and just response when things do not work out as anticipated or expected, and where the special bond of trust is put at risk.

Final Thoughts

In many ways, this book represents a resurfacing, refocusing, contextualisation and operationalisation of several first principles of quality thinking that have been lost in much of healthcare's adoption and spread of quality improvement. In the previous two decades where quality improvement has risen in prominence, this has been an unintentional missed opportunity by those agencies and departments tasked with identifying innovations in the service. In the early 2000s we were part of that missed opportunity and this book also represents our reflection on that time; a time where spread was all important and thus simpler tools and methods were prioritised. The net result was that those programmes aimed to make the current system of work better, rather than to fundamentally question it and do better things.

These principles have always been there if looked for carefully enough, but they have not been widely adopted and understood at a leadership or operational level. Perhaps some of the reason is that they don't offer quick clean solutions or engaging tools; they don't lend themselves to quick spread. They require people to consider them in context, reflect and think deeply about the tensions they surface. To be able to question the work in this way requires time and humility – factors that are scarce in many settings.

In a comparable manner, this book is a response to the marginalisation of difficult messages that surface when we do question the work. For our system of care to achieve greater quality and productivity, the work often fundamentally needs to change. This means that systems of leadership and governance need to change alongside it. This requires letting go of much of what is familiar and moves leaders into a space of surfacing and working with tensions, complexity and paradox, rather than implementing clean solutions and neat processes. Against this backdrop, much of this book tries to make this adoption of core quality thinking easier by providing principles which we believe help busy but curious leaders question the work.

Throughout this book, we have invited a great deal of consideration of possibilities and potential solutions to the issues under discussion. They provide a basis for curiosity and inquiry into the human condition, as propositions for exploration rather than aiming for definite answers through traditional scientific method. We recognise that no amount of knowledge or understanding will ever be enough to "solve" many of the issues under discussion, which are by their very nature emergent, dynamic and deeply embedded in the complexity of everyday relationships, enacted and adapted at a local level.

As a reader, we hope you have experienced an invitation to adopt a position of curious inquiry, which is more tentative and which holds ideas more lightly as reasonable possibilities, which might help us to "know how to go on" in specific situations. We hope that you have also understood that what we are asking is for you to question – and potentially reject – some of the "grand narratives" and "absolute truths" about the healthcare world, which we believe play a significant role in replicating some of our existing problematic ways of working.

We offer these ideas as "food for thought" and as a deliberate counteragent to the anti-intellectual, tool-driven, mechanistic approach that still dominates much of healthcare quality improvement work. Whilst enticing to those who promote them, they tend to invite reductionism, the atomisation of complex issues, the dismissal of shaping ideologies, and lead to simplistic and unsustainable outcomes.

We certainly don't promise a panacea, but instead invite curiosity and aim to stimulate dialogue. This book certainly won't solve the problems of healthcare quality, but we hope it will be a valuable and provocative contribution to the debate.

Index

Page numbers in *italic* indicate figures and in **bold** indicate tables.